Medical Technologies and the Life World

Although the use of new technologies in healthcare and medicine is generally seen as beneficial, there has been little analysis of the impact of such technologies on people's lives and understandings of health and illness. This book explores how new technologies not only provide hope for cure and well-being, but also introduce new ethical dilemmas and raise questions about the 'natural' body.

Focusing on the ways new medical technologies intervene into our lives and affect our notions of health, illness and normality, *Medical Technologies and the Life World* explores:

- how medical technologies are understood and used by practitioners in everyday clinical practice
- how medical technologies, and the ways they are used, are understood by patients in clinical encounters, and more generally in the context of their everyday lives
- how results or outcomes of these technologies are communicated in various clinical settings
- how new technologies can alter our notions of health and illness and create 'new illness'.

Written by authors with backgrounds in sociology, social psychology, philosophy, communication studies and nursing, this book discusses new technologies from a 'life-world' perspective. It is based on empirical studies of the use of various medical technologies and is essential reading for students and academics of medical sociology, health sciences, and science and technology studies.

Sonja Olin Lauritzen is Professor at the Department of Education, Stockholm University, Sweden.

Lars-Christer Hydén is Professor at the Department of Communication Studies, Linköping University, Sweden.

Critical Studies in Health and Society
Series Editors Simon J. Williams and Gillian Bendelow

This major new international book series takes a critical look at health in a rapidly changing social world. The series includes theoretically sophisticated and empirically informed contributions on cutting-edge issues from leading figures within the sociology of health and allied disciplines and domains. Other titles in the series include:

Contesting Psychiatry
Social movements in mental health
Nick Crossley

Men and their Health
Masculinity, social inequality and health
Alan Dolan

Lifestyle in Medicine
Gary Easthope and Emily Hansen

Medical Sociology and Old Age
Towards a sociology of health in later life
Paul Higgs and Ian Rees Jones

Emotional Labour in Health Care
Catherine Theodosius

Written in a lively, accessible and engaging style, with many thought-provoking insights, the series will cater to a truly interdisciplinary audience of researchers, professionals, practitioners and policy makers with an interest in health and social change.

Those interested in submitting proposals for single or co-authored, edited or co-edited volumes should contact the series editors, Simon J. Williams (s.j.williams@warwick.ac.uk) and Gillian Bendelow (g.a.bendelow@sussex. ac.uk).

Medical Technologies and the Life World

The social construction of normality

Edited by
Sonja Olin Lauritzen and
Lars-Christer Hydén

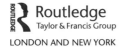

LONDON AND NEW YORK

First published 2007
by Routledge
2 Park Square, Milton Park, Abingdon, Oxon OX14 4RN

Simultaneously published in the USA and Canada
by Routledge
270 Madison Ave, New York, NY 10016

Routledge is an imprint of the Taylor & Francis Group, an informa business

Typeset in Sabon by
HWA Text and Data Management, Tunbridge Wells
Printed and bound in Great Britain by
The Cromwell Press, Trowbridge, Wiltshire

British Library Cataloguing in Publication Data
A catalogue record for this book is available from the British Library

Library of Congress Cataloging-in-Publication Data
Medical technologies and the life world / [edited by] Sonja Olin Lauritzen
    and Lars-Christer Hydén
      p.; cm. – (Critical studies in health and society)
    Includes bibliographical references and index.
    1. Medical ethics   2. Medical technology – Moral and ethical aspects
    I. Olin Lauritzen, Sonja.   II. Hydén, Lars-Christer, 1954–   III. Series
    [DNLM: 1. Sociology, Medical – methods.   2. Technology, Medical
    – ethics.   3. Clinical Medicine – methods.   4. Ethics, Medical
    WA 31 M48935 2007]
    R274.M43 2007
    610.28–dc22   2006017546

ISBN10: 0–415–36433–7 (hbk)
ISBN10: 0–415–36434–5 (pbk)
ISBN10: 0–203–01545–2 (ebk)

ISBN13: 978–0–415–36433–1 (hbk)
ISBN13: 978–0–415–36434–8 (pbk)
ISBN13: 978–0–203–01545–2 (ebk)

Contents

Contributors

Anette Forss, PhD, has a background in social anthropology as well as nursing, and is a researcher and lecturer at the Division of Nursing at the Karolinska Institute, Huddinge, Sweden. She has a research interest in biomedical technology, medical regimes, construction of normality and deviance in medical practice, and in people's experiences of medical interventions.

Susanne Georgsson Öhman, PhD, RN and RM, is a researcher at the Department of Neurobiology, Health Care Sciences and Society at the Karolinska Institute, Huddinge, Sweden. She has a research interest in reproductive health, particularly women's reactions and experiences of prenatal screening and diagnostics.

Lars-Christer Hydén, PhD (Psychology), is a professor at the Department of Communication, Linköping University, Sweden. His research area is language and social interaction, with a special focus on narrative.

Ann-Cristine Jonsson, PhD, is Public Health Planning Officer within the area of sexual and reproductive health at the Swedish National Institute of Public Health. Her research interests deal with the everyday understanding of preventive medicine and medical technology, and the construction of health and normality in the clinical situation.

Antje Lumma, PhD candidate at Linköping University, Sweden, has a university degree in psychology ('Diplompsychologe', Dipl. Psych.) from Marburg, Germany. Her doctoral thesis deals with medical students' attitudes towards learning in small groups, particularly learning to communicate with patients.

Sonja Olin Lauritzen, PhD, is a professor at the Department of Education, Stockholm University. Her research interests are in the field of everyday understanding of health and illness, and in the construction of normality and deviance in the interface between everyday and professional discourses.

Sissel Saltvedt, MD, PhD, is an obstetrician at the Department of Obstetrics and Gynaecology, South General Hospital in Stockholm. Her research interest is in reproductive health and prenatal diagnostics.

Fredrik Svenaeus, PhD, is a professor at the Centre for Practical Knowledge, Södertörn University College. His current research interests are philosophy of medicine and bioethics, especially issues of normality in connection with implementation of new health care technologies and therapies. Svenaeus has mainly worked within the research traditions of phenomenology and hermeneutics, with an emphasis on philosophy of practice and ethics of health care professions.

Gunilla Tegern, PhD, is a senior lecturer at the Department of Health and Society, Linköping University. Her research interests are in the field of health, illness and health care from an everyday perspective with a special focus on the mutual influence between medical thought and common sense.

Kristin Zeiler, PhD, is a researcher at the Department of Health and Society, Linköping University. Her research areas are bioethics and feminist ethics as well as global and theological ethics.

1 Medical technologies, the life world and normality

An introduction

Sonja Olin Lauritzen and
Lars-Christer Hydén

In recent years, the role and social impact of medical technologies, in the clinical world as well in the everyday world of patients, has become a topic in social science, and particularly so in the sociology of health and illness. The development of 'new' medical technologies has triggered a debate about the consequences of medical technologies for definitions of health, illness and disability as well as our understandings of the body. Some medical technologies, such as genetic diagnostic testing, have the capacity to detect deviance or disease before we ourselves are aware of any signs of illness. Others, for example the ultra-sound scan or magnetic resonance imaging, offer more and more sophisticated methods to 'look into the body' and have the capacity to produce new images of the body. Medical technology is used also to enhance health and normality, for example in plastic surgery or SSRI medication, to mention just two examples.

The use of these and other medical technologies may provide 'a fountain of hope' but they also introduce new ethical dilemmas and raises questions about the 'natural' body and about how the line is drawn between health and illness (Williams 1997). As a consequence, they may also create 'new illness'. The body, Brown and Webster argue, has become more 'available, accessible, mobile and dematerialized' (2004: 17). This, in turn, raises questions as to whether or not medical technology is engendering 'a crisis of meaning surrounding the human body at the turn of the 21st Century' (Williams 1997: 1047).

The introduction of new medical technologies as routine or large-scale practices in health care will confront an increasing number of patients, as well as practitioners, with new information about the body, new choices and decisions to be taken. Of particular interest is the role technology plays in the classificatory system of medicine that defines normality and abnormality. Within the sociology of health and illness, the impact of medical technologies has been discussed in relation to the organization of health care, professional practice as well as patients' experiences (Heath *et al.* 2003). However, there is still a lack of knowledge about these rapidly changing scenarios in health care and the ways medical technologies intervene into our lives and affect our ideas about the healthy and the ill body, our self-identity and relations to others.

This book addresses the social impact of medical technologies, more specifically how they feature in clinical practice and the meaning they take on in the life world of practitioners as well as patients, particularly in the construction of normality and deviance. The authors have differing backgrounds in sociology, social psychology, communication studies, phenomenology and the nursing sciences, but are in this book united in a 'life-world' perspective. Based on empirical studies of the use of various medical technologies, and how they are interpreted and communicated in different professional and everyday contexts, the following themes will be addressed theoretically as well as empirically:

- How are medical technologies understood and used by practitioners in everyday clinical practice?
- How are results or outcomes of these technologies communicated in various clinical settings?
- How are medical technologies, and the ways they are used, understood by patients in clinical encounters and more generally in the context of their everyday lives?
- What is the impact of these technologies on people's notions of health, illness and normality?

The focus of this book is not primarily on the sociology of medical technologies 'per se' – this has been discussed elsewhere (see for instance Elston 1997; Heath *et al.* 2003; Brown and Webster 2004). Our focus is on how medical technologies are understood from a life-world perspective, what consequences it has for communication between medical professionals and patient, and finally how ideas about normality and abnormality are affected – issues that we want to explore more fully in the chapters that follow. However, we first want to address the question of 'what are medical technologies?' and in what sense some technologies are regarded as 'new', as a back-drop to our inquiries into people's experiences and understanding of such technologies.

Medical technologies

Medical technologies can be described and categorized in different ways. Brown and Webster (2004) discuss medical technologies as related to different fields of medical development. '*Information and communication technologies*', such as the use of the Internet to access medical information as well as social support, the electronic patient record, sonography and telemedicine, are characterized by the way they disconnect the experiencing patient and the corporal body from the medical information about the patient. Visual images and other data produced by the technology can be communicated, electronically or otherwise, world-wide and independently of the individual patient. In this sense, these technologies can be said to be reordering the relationship between practitioners and patients.

Technologies that can be related to *'new biologies'*, for example trans-species transplantation and various types of gene technology, offer new possibilities in the prediction and prevention of future disease, but also generate new risk identities and uncertainties. Another set of technologies create 'cyborg' hybrids or *'assemblages'* in bringing together machine and body tissue. One example is 'regenerative medicine' producing artificial body parts and intra-body instruments. These technologies thus raise a series of 'difficult and challenging questions concerning the character of our human/ non-human identity' (Brown and Webster 2004: 2).

The consequences of medical technologies for medical practice as well as for patients can of course be described in different ways depending on the perspective and purpose of the analysis. Today, there is much debate about *'new'* medical technology that can generate more paradigmatic shifts in medicine and in the relationship between professionals and patients (or patients-to-be). The development of increasingly sophisticated optical devices (for example the X-ray and ultrasound technology) has opened up radically new ways to 'look into the body'. The 'new genetics' has created new possibilities to 'look into the future', as it is used for example in diagnostic situations. Another aspect of the novelty of medical technology is that the *role* of technology in medicine can change as development in medical knowledge and medical training is increasingly defined in technical rather than professional terms something that in turn may affect the relationship between expert and lay discourse.

Even if much of the modern medical technology is presented as new, some technologies can rather be seen as 'more of the same', as applied in new clinical contexts or as presented as new by those who develop or use the technology. Also, technology can be combined in 'clusters' that will be new, including mundane and routine uses of medical technologies (Brown and Webster 2004). One example is antenatal care where new components of advanced technology, such as ultrasound screening of the foetus, are added to a well-established routine health surveillance programme. Furthermore, medical technologies are found in highly specialized medicine, for example specialist clinics for genetic counselling or diagnostics, as well as in routine primary health care, such as the regular Pap-smear screening of all women above a certain age. In Timmermans and Berg's words, 'medicine forms an archaeology of layer upon layer of technologies from the most mundane band-aids and pencils to sophisticated machines such as MRIs and artificial hearts, from virtually neutral infusion pumps to highly symbolic procedures and devices such as the drug Viagra or genetic tests' (2003: 99).

How are we to make sense of these medical technologies (and the debates they trigger)? One important point of departure is that medical technology always appears, and is understood, in a context, and thus cannot 'speak' entirely for itself. It takes on meaning in the social, cultural and clinical context where it is used, and it therefore makes sense to look at the development of medical technology *and* the way it is applied in clinical practice. This means that it is necessary to understand 'how the technology is enveloped in practice and practical circumstance' (Heath *et al.* 2003: 78).

In a review of publications on technology and medical practice over the last 25 years in the journal *Sociology of Health and Illness*, Heath *et al.* (2003) draw the conclusion that these publications reveal how 'practical circumstances and contexts in healthcare bear upon the ways in which these tools and technologies come to be perceived and understood' and that the character of these technologies is 'determined by participants themselves within the practicalities of their ordinary lives' (ibid: 83). Also, the features and meaning of medical technology are dependent on, shaped and mediated through social interaction in clinical practice. At the heart of this question is the issue of the professional–patient relationship. As Brown and Webster argue, the '*immediacy of the clinical encounter is the medium through which the technology is experienced*, whether as a one-off or a multiple series of interactive events' (2004: 168, italics in original).

This 'points to the importance of placing the practical circumstances, the situation in which tools and technologies are deployed, at the forefront of analytical agenda' (Heath *et al.* 2003: 83) and the importance of taking account of the local, the routine, practical and 'indigenous' use of the technologies in everyday practice within specific courses of action and interaction, something that is still largely unexplored. Furthermore, medical technologies appear in a range of medical contexts, and medicine is in turn embedded in wider social and cultural processes that involve understandings of health, illness and the body. Important components of these understandings have to do with how people are inclined to question medical knowledge and practice at the same time as they look to medicine and medical technology for new hopes for remedies (Williams and Calnan 1996).

In this book we will address medical technology as it is used in clinical practice, and explore the meanings medical technologies take on for the patient as well as the health professional. To be able to look further into these issues, we first want to briefly discuss the notion of the life-world perspective, and how this perspective has been adapted to the study of health and illness.

The life world and the world of medicine

In the social science exploration of the ways people in the Western cultures relate to their illnesses, a recurrent theme through the decades has been the relationship between, on the one hand, the patient, her body, experiences and management of illness, and on the other hand, the needs of the medical system to fit the patient and her ailments into the administrative, cognitive and procedural organization of modern medicine; that is, the way the ill *person* is transformed into a legitimate *patient* in the medical health care system.

One central problem to researchers in this field is the meaning and consequences of the modern big and complex health care organizations and systems. One of the most important features of these organizations and systems is the increasingly specialized medical knowledge and technology and its tight connection to specific professions and professional groups (specialized medical doctors and registered nurses, and various equally specialized paramedical professions).

The potential conflict between the experiences and knowledge of the patient and the health care system has been conceptualized as a conflict between the patient's *life world* and *the world of medicine*. These two central concepts – the life world and the world of medicine – go back to ideas introduced by the philosopher Edmund Husserl in his book *The Crisis of European Sciences* (1970). Husserl's idea was that all our human knowledge is built on the lived everyday experience of the world – what he called the 'life world'. Due to practical needs and problems we start to contemplate not only the world but our own experience of the world. We do this for instance through an abstracting attitude towards our own experience – that is, we become self-reflective. Husserl used the example of geometry, and argued that we, as human beings, over time have learnt to abstract more general and recurrent spatial forms from the everyday practical experience of the shapes of things in the world. As a consequence everyday knowledge is to be regarded as a prerequisite for scientific knowledge. In a similar way, the philosopher Georges Canguilhem (1991) has pointed out that the everyday experience of the body, as well as its ailments, is a prerequisite for the development of scientific medical knowledge about various diseases.

The ideas of Edmund Husserl were adapted to the field of social science first of all by Alfred Schutz (1962) and Harold Garfinkel (1967). They argued that everyday world knowledge could be characterized by its uncritical, practical-pragmatic and taken-for-granted attitude towards both the world and experience. The knowledge of science on the other hand, is characterized by opposite qualities: a critical, theoretical and systematic attitude towards phenomena and experience.

These concepts were used by the social psychologist Elliot Mishler when writing about the different attitudes of patients and doctors in medical interviews in his book *The Discourse of Medicine* (1984). More specifically, patients and doctors relate to the complaints and problems that the patient presents in the medical interview in two different ways. Elliot Mishler argued that in medical interviews, two voices, that is, two ways of relating to and talking about bodily problems could be discerned: what he called the voice of the life world and the voice of medicine. These two voices will sometimes be in conflict in the medical encounter; the voice of the life world struggles against the voice of medicine in order to be heard and recognized by the doctor (see Mishler 2005 for an update of his views). The idea of the two worlds are then used in order to point out that patients and doctors have different kinds of knowledge and attitudes towards bodies and illnesses; and also that often a conflict or struggle between these two worlds is manifested in the encounter between the patient on the one hand and the doctor and the health care system on the other hand. Here, a special problem is how the voice of the patient is subordinated by the medical voice as the life world experiences and knowledge is transformed into the language and procedures of the medical world. Today, however, there is more discussion about the voice of the patient not only as subordinated to medicine, but as knowledgeable and articulated as for example in 'expert patients'.

The concepts of the life world and the medical world have been used to relate the different types of experience, knowledge and attitudes to each other in a dynamic way, and to discuss their potential conflicts and transformations. In many ways it has been an alternative to the concepts of lay and expert knowledge that establishes two realms of knowledge where expert knowledge is being transformed and adopted by lay knowledge, although always superior. The concept of a life world has also been used by researchers who want to explore the experiences of the ill and suffering person, particularly within phenomenological research traditions (see for instance Toombs 1992).

Medical technology has a rationality, that is an aim and a working logic, which has developed out of the world of medicine. Technological devices have been constructed in order to solve problems and serve purposes that are primarily part of the medical practice. They help and enhance medical professionals in their work (cf. Mol 2002). In many cases this rationality fits into the everyday rationality of patients: patients want the medical professionals to help them remediate their diseases. In these cases medical technology can be taken as a self-evident and given part of medical practice, even if the patient does not necessarily understand the workings of the technology. In other cases problems emerge when the medical rationality does not immediately correspond to or is not possible to translate into the logic of everyday life. This is the case for instance with many of the life-supportive systems used in order to help patients live on, even when they are severely ill (Robillard 1999). Medical technology has in these cases its own rationality, which does not automatically correspond to the life world rationality of the patient.

In other cases, medical technology can raise problems that are not part of the medical world but are part of the everyday world. A typical example is the type of moral problems that various types of screening technologies (ultrasound, genetic screening) result in. When some sort of deviance is found, the patient has to make a decision, for instance about having an abortion or not. The moral problem is here part of the patient's life world, his or her hopes and expectations, and can only be answered in that context. A similar situation emerges when medical technology produces unwarranted information as part of an examination, as for instance when parents learn the sex of their expected baby at the ultrasound scan, without having asked for or wanted this information.

Communication in the clinical encounter

As we have already mentioned, the clinical encounter is the medium through which the medical technology is experienced by the individual. Traditionally, most of the research on communication between patients and medical practitioners has focused on the medical interview, especially interviews in general practice (Atkinson 1995; Hydén and Mishler 1999). This may be natural due to the fact that probably most encounters between patients and medical professionals take place in general practice, and that this is the type of encounter that most people are involved in. Studies of communication have thus largely focused on the prototypical encounter in general practice and on the dialogue between 'the doctor' and 'the patient' (ibid).

However, clinical practice has changed, not least due to the development of medical technology, and so have the conditions for communication between the different parties involved. These changes have to do with, among other things, new divisions of tasks between primary health care and specialized or hospital-based clinical practice. The development of, for example, methods for various types of screening, as well as new non-invasive examinations, have made it possible to carry out more 'advanced' tasks on patients on a regular basis in primary health care. Also, medical knowledge has, as a result, become even more specialized, and hosts different specialized professions in addition to the medical doctor, such as the laboratory assistants, specialists in physics, etc., who have increasingly become important in medical work. As a consequence, communicative co-ordination between different medical specialists, and also paramedical staff, is needed in medical work. Also team organization, bringing various professions together in clinical work with a joint clinical goal, has become more common in medical work, leading to more complex forms of communication (especially talk in groups, see for instance Linell 1998).

Through the changes in medical technology, as well as in the professional organizations and tasks, the relationship between practitioners and patients has become more complicated and organizationally mediated. The relationship between the individual patient and the individual doctor, and traditional dyadic forms of communication, is replaced with multiple relations: between those parts of the patient's body that are represented by technology, such as a lab sample or an X-ray image, and between various medical professionals encountering and analysing these representations. Paul Atkinson argues that the patient's 'body is dispersed through multiple sites of investigation throughout [the] organizational complexity' of the modern hospital (Atkinson 1995: 61). To this could be added that the medical profession as well is dispersed throughout the organizational complexity resulting in multiple relations between the patient, his or her body and various specialized professionals. Some of these relations are instantiated as actual face-to-face encounters, others take place in cyberspace or inter-professional conversations with the patient as the absent-present 'Third'.

Modern medicine has in many ways widened the traditional notion of diseases as being located *in* the body (Armstrong 2002). Today it is generally acknowledged that diseases in many cases also include the patient's life and lifestyle, and that the disease has consequences in the life of the patient in ways that potentially affect the treatment. This means that medical professionals have to talk about areas that are generally associated with the life world of the patient; and in ways that give the medical professional the possibility to both advise and negotiate these matters (see Sarangi *et al.* 2005).

In order to be able to advise patients, for instance about genetic information, or to influence patients to change their lifestyle, it can be seen as necessary not only to talk *to* the patients, but above all *with* the patients. This would mean that the medical professional has to invite the patient into the medical encounter and be able to respond to the patient in ways that include the patient and his or her perspective in the conversation. Also, in contemporary society, people have vast possibilities to access medical information, for instance through the Internet, and will bring this kind of information *to* the encounter with the doctor.

These changes make it important to examine the ways in which medical technologies feature in clinical encounters. We could think of at least three ways this can happen. First, in some cases the medical encounter becomes directly mediated by technology in the sense that the medical professional uses a technological device during the physical examination. This is the case for example in the ultrasound examination or the PET scan. The technological device becomes an integrated part of the ongoing clinical encounter and has to be explained and reckoned with in many ways.

Second, medical technology can also produce results that are used in the clinical encounter. Referring to lab reports in the clinical encounter is not something new, but the extent and importance of these types of results and reports have probably increased. It means that the doctor has access to information that the patient generally does not have; and if the patient has access, he or she can most probably not interpret it without professional assistance (unless the patient is an 'expert patient'). Much of this information can be abstract and does not easily translate into the context of the everyday world. This creates challenges for the practitioners to find ways to communicate the meaning of medical technologies and the information about the individual patient that is produced, as well as challenges related to how information from medical technologies can be 'translated' into medical advice that makes sense to the patient.

Finally, when the information produced by the technology is communicated, some of this will have consequences for the patient's lifestyle, hopes for the future and understanding of their own bodies. That is, some information will raise problems in the everyday life of the patient, but not necessarily in the medical world. Results from tests and examinations can have consequences for the individual patient and his or her relatives, in the sense that it changes the life course or the possibilities in life for the individual. Other types of information put a demand on the patient and his or her relatives to make decisions about for instance having children, or whether to reveal knowledge about a genetic risk to their children. As a consequence, medical professionals often have to be able to take part in these types of discussions, and try to help patients and their relatives to explore possibilities and to reach a decision. This is not something new in medicine, but has probably become a more general problem, affecting many more medical professionals in various specialities – and their patients.

The construction of normality

As we have argued, medical technology and the results these technologies produce, can take on different meanings in the world of medicine and the life world. One important and intriguing question has to do with the role medical technology plays in relation to the process of defining normality and abnormality and the (changing) boundaries in between.

The modern usage of the word 'normal', Ian Hacking (1990) argues, evolved in the nineteenth century in a medical context, more precisely in pathology. 'The normal was one of a pair. Its opposite was the pathological and for a short time its domain was chiefly medical' (Hacking 1990: 160). Something was normal when it was not associated with a pathological organ, and the normal was thus secondary, the opposite of the pathological. Hacking (ibid.) describes how this then was 'turned around' (by Comte) and the pathological became secondary, characterized in terms of deviation from the normal, or from 'the normal state'. Importantly, pathology was not understood as a different kind from the normal; 'nature makes no jumps' but passes from the normal to the pathological continuously, and the normal is the centre from which deviation departs. 'There is no pathological disturbance in itself, the abnormal can only be evaluated in terms of relationship' (Canguilhem 1991: 188).

One of the long-standing debates concerning the concept of normality has to do with the relationship between the normal and abnormal or pathological, more specifically *where* normal variation ends and abnormality begins. It has been argued that more attention should be given to variations of the normal. One interesting example is the way women's health and bodily processes have been treated as deviations from a norm based on the male body. The feminist biologist Linda Birke (1999) has pointed out that deviations from the normal could be understood as 'differences' rather that pathological, and that normality/abnormality then could be conceptualized as variations of the normal/deviations from the normal.

The concern with identification of pathology in the ill person which was at the heart of 'Hospital Medicine', was replaced by a concern with normal populations in twentieth-century 'Surveillance Medicine' (Armstrong 1995). A precondition of surveillance was the problematization of the normal. Within this medical paradigm, the distinct categories of healthy and ill are dissolved in an attempt to bring everyone within a network of visibility. The individual body is placed in a field that is not delineated by the absolute categories of normality and abnormality, but by the characteristics of the normal population. 'The new dimensionality of identity is to be found in the shift from a three-dimensional body as the locus of illness to the four-dimensional space of the time-community' (ibid.: 403). Illness is thus placed in a new temporal context, where risk factors are pointers to a potential yet unformed eventuality.

If we look at contemporary practice, the notions of normality, abnormality and a potential abnormality seem to take on different meanings in different contexts. In the *everyday practice of medicine*, health professionals draw on scientific definitions of normality as well as clinical experience and everyday knowledge. Notions of normality are shared with the local clinical community and communicated in clinical encounters with patients. Normality can be defined statistically or clinically, and is closely linked to the concepts of health and illness. Hoedemaekers and ten Have (1999) argue that in a non-scientific usage, health tends to be associated with normality (as an absence of disease or apparent pathology). Health, as adequate functioning and performance is also the state found in the majority of cases, and therefore considered normal. Disease is found in a smaller number of people, and tends to be connected with abnormality (1999: 539). However, it is not always clear whether the normal represents the state of the average person or an 'ideal type' in terms of optimal functioning, appearance or performance (or minimal functioning). 'The normal indicates how the organ or human body should function, it is the function which is desirable for all' (ibid.: 540). Thus, the ways the concepts of normality and abnormality are used in everyday clinical practice can be described as complex and problematic.

Today, medical technology increasingly plays an important role when abnormality is diagnosed and when potentially abnormal individuals are 'sorted out', as well as when efforts are made to enhance normality – and new methods that open up new possibilities and more precise methods are continuously introduced. Medical technology is used in clinical practice to diagnose abnormality, for example in prenatal diagnostics to identify foetuses with certain malformations or genes which will lead to future disease or disability. Technology is used in screening to 'sort out' individuals at high risk of having an abnormality, according to certain established criteria. However, the process by which these methods are applied and integrated in clinical practice are quite complex, and are in turn embedded in the local culture of the clinic with its particular rules, norms and traditions. The task of using medical technology, and interpreting and communicating the outcome in encounters with patients, is thus something that medical professionals 'learn' in the context of medical work. Of particular interest here is how these rules, norms and traditions have to be 'learned' by new members in clinical practice (Atkinson 1995).

In the *everyday life of the patient*, understandings of normality are embedded in the everyday knowledge that is constantly negotiated and developed in the interface between the expert and everyday world. One the one hand, empirical studies indicate that people seem to rely on the various notions of normality that are found in clinical practice; normality as the typical, as the average and as the desired. Hoedemaekers and ten Have argue that in everyday usage, 'the normal represents usualness: that which is familiar, habitual, common, found frequently, or in accordance with what can be expected' (1999: 539). The abnormal represents that which is considered different from what is usual. Also in the everyday context, the normal may become normative, particularly with reference to behaviour.

On the other hand, a typical pattern seems to be that normality, and risks of abnormality, is understood in a more binary way. It seems to be difficult to think of oneself in terms of a certain relative risk of abnormality. De Swaan (1990) argues that in cases of 'a small chance of a great misfortune' the odds will be known to some extent, but this 'does not establish the meaning of the early danger signals for the proto-patient and the doctor' (1990: 61). For the patient, results will always have to be translated into an all or nothing: as an individual, I am either sick or healthy (ibid). Patients do not typically conceptualize risk in terms of statistical probabilities, but rather as danger. In the process of making sense of this danger, they draw on ontological and cosmological assumptions and experiences in their life worlds (Lupton 1995).

This would indicate that *variations* in normality and deviance are (more) difficult to understand within a life-world perspective. Furthermore, people rather tend to see diagnostic tests and screening as a means to *confirm* normality, which has been demonstrated for instance in the field of reproductive health (Green 1990). Also when information about risk of abnormality is communicated in clinical encounters, the typical pattern of communication is to confirm normality and to use different rhetorical strategies, by practitioners as well as patients, to avoid or down-play the issue of abnormality (Bredmar and Linell 1999).

Information about risk of abnormality is often presented as abstract figures, scores or graphs, that have to be *re-interpreted* by the individual to make sense in the context of her own life world (Lupton 1995). A calculated risk for a specific abnormality, a risk figure or a curve on a chart, has to be understood *as something* (familiar to the individual) to make sense (Adelswärd and Sachs 1996, Olin Lauritzen and Sachs 2001). Furthermore, everyday reasoning is also characterized by the way people draw on different explanations and ways of understanding the meaning of risk information, and are able to move in a flexible way between different interpretations, also contradictory ones (Davison *et al.* 1991).

Medical technologies can have intended as well as unintended social consequences. When people are faced with medical technology, and maybe particularly when new and yet unfamiliar technology is introduced, this will also draw people's attention to the possible abnormalities that the technologies are designed to detect or deal with, abnormalities that they might have been 'happily' unaware of until they are confronted with a new test, examination or a new possibility to enhance normality. This opens up new arenas and possibilities, but also new decisions to be taken. Some technologies also produce unwarranted information, in addition to the clinical purpose that they are used for. Ultrasound technology, for instance, can provide information about malformation, and the sex of the foetus, that is to date not included in the routine examination. In this and other clinical situations, unwarranted information may create dilemmas for the practitioner as well as for the patient. The practitioner will have to decide whether these findings should be communicated to the patient, and how. The patient will have to make sense of information he or she had not asked for and was unprepared for, information that might affect their thinking about the future and possible life course.

Of particular interest is the situation people find themselves in when technology is used not only to treat illness but also to enhance health. Once a technology exists, it can be used for different purposes and for a wider range of health problems. Today, there is an on-going discussion about new types of technology and medication that are applied in a range of situations, from treatment of illness to promotion of health. In the field of mental health, for instance, this development is addressed by Carl Elliott in his book *Better Than Well* (2003) in relation to the way medication, such as SSRIs, is used in contemporary society, not only to treat mental illness but also to enhance wellbeing.

Medical technology thus confronts professionals as well as patients with new decisions to be taken, and also new uncertainties. As the body has become a 'project' open to intervention and control, an important aspect of medical technology is inherently tied to 'the manufacture and circulation of hopes and promises' (Brown and Webster 2004: 180). The flip-side of these hopes and promises is the issue of trust and uncertainty. As Zygmunt Bauman (1993) argues, characteristic of modernity is our sense of uncertainty in the face of a range of competing choices for action. From this point of view, medical technology can be seen as 'symbolically expressing' the dilemmas of life in an increasingly uncertain age (Williams 1997: 1048).

The scope of this book

In this book, we will address medical technology as related to the life world: how the life world enters into medical practice and into practitioners' dealings with medical technologies and the ways medical technologies have an impact on the life world, with a focus on how normality is constructed in these processes.

We will first address clinical practice and the ways professionals 'learn', or are 'socialized', to carry out their professional tasks and how patients and bodies become categorized in the clinical context. Then, we will look into patients' experiences and understandings of their encounters with the medical world and medical technology, and their understanding of themselves and their bodies as healthy and normal – or not. Throughout the book, we will draw on examples of technology that, in different ways, intervene into the everyday lives of people and (potentially) have an impact on their life course and expectations for the future: reproductive health technologies, technologies for early detection of serious or life-threatening diseases and technologies that will intervene into the well-being of individuals.

All the chapters in this book are based on studies carried out in Sweden. This means that the empirical studies we discuss are set within the same general frame in terms of culture and health care system. Even if some aspects of this background might be specific to Sweden, such as details of the health care organization, the issues we want to discuss in this book are related to experiences and dilemmas in the use of medical technology that are not limited to national contexts but more general and shared in modern medicine.

In Chapter 2, Lars-Christer Hydén and Antje Lumma discuss the development and use of communicative technology and ideology in modern medicine with a focus on the relationship between the medical doctor and the patient. Communicative strategies and practices are seen as a type of social technology alongside other types of 'technical' technologies most commonly associated with medicine. Modern medical practice is among other things characterized by the fact that medical doctors have to investigate not only the bodily interior of patients, but also the social and moral space of patients. This means that medical professionals have to be able to talk with patients in many different types of medical contexts and also be able to talk about topics that are related to the patient's life world. In many medical educational programs, learning to talk with patients has the status of an independent course. In this chapter, examples from one such course are used in order to illustrate problems in learning to talk with patients.

In Chapter 3, Anette Forss discusses the ways assessment of normality and abnormality is carried out in everyday laboratory work, based on a one-year-long ethnographic study conducted at two cytology laboratories. As the interpreter of the Pap smear, a screening test which has become routine in health care for women, the cytodiagnostician has a central role in determining the need for further investigation of cellular abnormalities, something that has implications for both patients and professionals. In the chapter, the daily work of analysing and classifying cells down the microscope is described and analysed. Drawing on a theoretical framework on visualization and classification, it is argued that screening cytology, including the Pap smear, can be seen as (em)bodied seeing. The biological maps of cells and cultural notions are mobilized and intertwined by the cytodiagnostician when interpreting cells, and the study reveals that cytodiagnosticians are highly aware of this interpretative nature of cytological assessments. In conclusion, it is argued that living people and living organisms do not form mutually exclusive realms in cytological assessments.

The ways in which health professionals reflect on their work in the 'sorting out' of deviation from normality is discussed also in Chapter 4. In this chapter Kristin Zeiler explores a case of diagnostic technology in reproductive health care, the pre-implantantation genetic diagnosis (PGD). The availability and use of assisted conception technologies combined with PGD evoke moral, social and existential questions. When PGD is discussed among health professionals and scientists, a number of stories are also told in which interpretations of disease, choice and normality are combined and re-combined in different ways. Three major types of stories or narratives are discussed in this chapter: *narratives of life with genetic disease*, *narratives of progress* and *narratives of ambivalence*. Interpretations of disease, choice and normality are, in a variety of ways, components of the fabric of these narratives, and they are used in the construction of a certain logic – as well as in the questioning of this logic – within and throughout the different narratives.

Technology in reproductive health is addressed also in Chapter 5, more precisely the routine ultrasound scan in maternity health care. In this chapter, Ann-Cristine Jonsson analyses the ways normality is communicated in regular ultrasound examinations of healthy pregnant women. The shimmering image on the ultrasound screen does not speak for itself, it has to be interpreted as the examination is being carried out. Ann-Cristine Jonsson explores this process of interpretation with a focus on the midwife's professional perspective as well as the parent's everyday perspective. The analysis reveals a process of communication where a range of strategies are used to confirm the normality of the expected baby – strategies that can be understood as ways to deal with a medical technology that confronts all parents-to-be with images of their unborn baby. It is argued that this technology 'forces' the parents to make sense of the visual images of the expected baby in a dialogue with the practitioner – and that they are thus forced to a reflexivity concerning the pregnancy, the baby and their future family.

The ultrasound scan is discussed again in Chapter 6. The scan is today part of the health surveillance of all pregnant women in most Western countries, and familiar to most of those concerned. At the same time, the ultrasound technology has become more sophisticated and offers possibilities to detect an increasing range of abnormalities in the foetus. One of the recent developments is ultrasound nuchal translucency screening for early detection of Down's syndrome. In this chapter Sonja Olin Lauritzen, Susanne Georgsson Öhman and Sissel Saltvedt explore women's experiences of false positive results of being at high risk after this screening. The analysis focuses on how the women try to make sense of the high risk information after the ultrasound scan and how they interpret the high risk figure, as well as the women's reflections on the normality of the baby-to-be. Of particular interest is how the screening, and the high risk information indicating a possible abnormality, seems to interrupt the 'normal' pregnancy and create difficulties for the women to return to this 'normal state' even long after confirmation of a normal foetus.

In Chapter 7, Gunilla Tegern discusses some of the impacts of advances in medical imaging technology, more specifically the magnetic resonance imaging scan. This technology can provide increasingly detailed information about intracranial aneurysms, information that can save lives, but also unwarranted information about so-called 'cold aneurysms' in people who see themselves as healthy. In this chapter, the author analyses people's experiences of a ruptured aneurysm and of unexpectedly being diagnosed with a 'cold aneurysm' presented in illness narratives on an Internet site. The focus of the analysis is here on the meaning of the intracranial aneurysm, and on the social representation of this condition that people draw on when trying to describe and understand their own experiences: the representation of a 'ticking bomb'. An important element in these narratives is how people try to come to terms with what it means to be living with the risk of a potentially life-threatening condition, without any symptoms, and how the self in this process comes to the forefront as a more or less permanent thematic object of attention.

A different type of technology is discussed in Chapter 8. During the 1990s the prescription of anti-depressive pharmaceutics, such as SSRIs, increased rapidly. Fredrik Svenaeus raises the question of how we can understand this SSRI revolution. How should we listen to Prozac, as the title of Peter Kramer's much-read book of 1994 urges us to do? An attempt is made to show how the philosophical tradition of phenomenology can pave the way for a better understanding of the issues involved in both the development of this technology and the pro–contra debates surrounding it. Three types of phenomena, characteristic of depression and anxiety disorders – painful feelings, problems with engagement in the world, and altered embodiment – are scrutinized in order to explore the realms of normal and abnormal being-in-the-world, mainly with the aid of the philosophy of Martin Heidegger. In addition to this, the concept of normality itself is subjected to a phenomenological analysis.

Through the different examples presented in this book we hope to shed more light on the impact of medical technologies, as they are used and communicated in clinical practice. More specifically, we would argue, the variety of the pieces of research that are discussed can help us to a more profound understanding of how the life world enters into the use of medical technologies, and how medical technologies are understood and their use intervenes into the life worlds of people. Finally, we hope this book will contribute to the emergent discussion about medical technologies and the ways they are understood and experienced by people within and outside the medical professions.

References

Adelswärd, V. and Sachs, L. (1996) 'A nurse in preventive work: dilemmas of health information talks', *Scandinavian Journal of Caring Science*, 10: 45–52.

Armstrong, D. (1995) 'The rise of surveillance medicine', *Sociology of Health and Illness*, 17: 393–404.

Armstrong, D. (2002) *A New History of Identity: A Sociology of Medical Knowledge*, London: Palgrave.

Atkinson, P. (1995) *Medical Talk and Medical Work: The Liturgy of the Clinic*, London: Sage.

Bauman, Z. (1993) *Modernity and Ambivalence*, Cambridge: Polity Press.

Birke, L. (1999) *Feminism and the Biological Body*, Edinburgh: Edinburgh University Press.

Bredmar, M. and Linell, P. (1999) 'Reconfirming normality: the construction of reassurance in talks between midwives and expectant mothers', in S. Sarangi and C. Roberts (eds) *Talk, Work and Institutional Order*, Berlin: Mouton de Gruyter.

Brown, N. and Webster, A. (2004) *New Medical Technologies and Society: Reordering Life*, Cambridge: Polity Press.

Canguilhem, G. (1991) *The Normal and the Pathological*, New York: Zone Books.

Davison, C., Smith, G. and Frankel, S. (1991) 'Lay epidemiology and the prevention paradox: the implication of coronary candidacy for health education', *Sociology of Health and Illness*, 13: 1–19.

Elliot, C. (2003) *Better Than Well: American Medicine Meets the American Dream*, New York: Norton.

Elston, M.A. (ed.) (1997) *The Sociology of Medical Science and Technology*, Oxford: Blackwell.

Garfinkel, H. (1967) *Studies in Ethnomethodology*, New York: Prentice-Hall.

Green, J.M. (1990) 'Prenatal screening and diagnosis: some psychological and social issues', *British Journal of Obstetrics and Gynaecology*, 97: 1074–6.

Hacking, I. (1990) *The Taming of Chance*, Cambridge: Cambridge University Press.

Heath, C., Luff. P. and Sanchez Svensson, M. (2003) 'Technology and medical practice', *Sociology of Health and Illness*, 25: 75–96.

Hoedemaekers, R. and ten Have, H. (1999) 'The concept of abnormality in medical genetics', *Theoretical Medicine and Bioethics*, 20: 537–61.

Hydén, L.C. and Mishler, E.G. (1999) 'Medicine and language', *Annual Review of Applied Linguistics*, 19: 174–92.

Husserl, E. (1970) *The Crisis of European Sciences and Transcendental Phenomenology*, Evanston: Northwestern University Press.

Linell, P. (1998) 'Discourse across boundaries: On recontextualizations and the blending of voices in professional discourse', *Text*, 18: 143–57.

Lupton, D. (1995) *The Imperative of Health: Public Health and the Regulated Body*, London: Sage.

Mishler, E.G. (1984) *The Discourse of Medicine: Dialectics of Medical Interviews*, Norwood, NJ: Ablex.

Mishler, E.G. (2005) 'Patient stories, narratives of resistance and the ethics of humane care: a la recherche du temps perdu', *Health*, 9: 431–51.

Mol, A. (2002) *The Body Multiple: Ontology in Medical Practice*, Durham, NC: Duke University Press.

Olin Lauritzen, S. and Sachs, L. (2001) 'Normality, risk and the future: implicit communication of threat in health surveillance', *Sociology of Health and Illness*, 23: 497–516.

Robillard, A.B. (1999) *Meaning of a Diability: The Lived Experience of Paralysis*, Philadelphia, PA: Temple University Press.

Sarangi, S., Bennert, K., Howell, L., Clarke, A., Harper, P. and Gray, J. (2005) '(Mis)alignments in counselling for Huntington's disease predictive testing: clients' responses to reflective frames', *Journal of Genetic Counselling*, 14: 29–42.

Schutz, A. (1962) *Collected Papers, vol. I. The Problem of Social Reality*, Dordrecht: Kluwer Academic.

Swaan de, A. (1990) *The Management of Normality: Critical Essays on Health and Welfare*, London: Routledge.

Timmermans, S. and Berg, M. (2003) 'The practice of medical technology', *Sociology of Health and Illness*, 25: 97–114.

Toombs, S.K. (1992) *The Meaning of Illness: A Phenomenological Account of the Different Perspectives of Physician and Patient*, Dordrecht: Kluwer Academic.

Williams, S.J. (1997) 'Modern medicine and the "uncertain body": from corporeality to hyperreality?', *Social Science and Medicine*, 45: 1041–9.

Williams, S.J. and Calnan, M. (eds) (1996) *Modern Medicine. Lay Perspectives and Experiences*, London: UCL Press.

2 Learning to talk and talking about talk

Professional identity and communicative technology

*Lars-Christer Hydén and
Antje Lumma*

Introduction

During the last fifty years major changes have taken place in medical knowledge, treatment and care, as well as in its organization. These changes concern both the medical practices and the social and cultural conditions of the health care system.

David Mechanic, an American medical sociologist, points out that the transformation in medicine has come not only from the introduction of new drugs, imaging devices, surgical tools and other biomedical technologies, but also from 'changing social and organizational technologies' (Mechanic 2002). We would like to point out that one such new social technology is the development of communicative technologies for the dialogue between doctors and patients, especially in the medical interview.

We do not often think of communication and social and verbal interaction in terms of technology, and especially not in the medical setting where ideas like compassion and active listening are considered central. Nevertheless, not only can ways of talking be learnt, but ways of talking strategically can also be learnt. In this context we can think of technology as a set of strategies used in order to produce certain ends or attain certain goals. Not only do clinical professionals like medical doctors, psychologists, psychotherapists and social workers learn these types of communicative strategies, but lawyers, police officers and members of other professions do as well. They also learn to how to *violate* and strategically use everyday conventions of talk in order to be able to pursue their professional goals, irrespective of their own and their clients' 'true' motivations.

In this chapter we discuss the development and use of communicative technology in modern medicine, focusing on the relationship between the medical doctor and the patient. We are especially interested in factors both *inside* and *outside* medicine that have affected this development, as well as how medical students learn to use modern medical communicative technologies and ideologies. Modern medicine is characterized by new types of situations in which medical doctors investigate not only the inside of the body, but also the social and moral spaces in which bodies live. They do this in order to suggest a diagnosis and treatment (coronary diseases), help the patient to change his or her life (stop smoking) or make vital decisions (genetic counselling). The medical doctor has to be able to use and elicit all the various types of information that are medically needed and contribute information to individuals and families in order to help them make decisions. This means that medical doctors have to be able to talk with almost all kinds of patients in various medical contexts.

Formalizing certain basic interactional strategies as communicative skills and part of a communicative ideology makes it possible to learn, practise and account for these skills. But learning to communicate with patients also means changing attitudes towards oneself and others, and especially towards medical colleagues.

We illustrate and exemplify this development by using examples from a study of the long-term course in medical communication that is part of the educational programme for medical doctors at a Swedish university. We especially want to illustrate the ways medical students acquire a *professional* way of communicating with patients, and show what problems they encounter and which coping strategies they employ. That is, we want to show how they learn to implement and use the communicative technology and ideology taught during their medical training courses, and the effect this practice has on their identities as medical doctors.

The changing medical field

The relationship between medical doctor and patient and the norms and ideals that guide and control this relationship are affected by a host of conditions both internal and external to medicine. These include the development of new medical technologies (Conrad 2005), changes having to do with the position of patients *vis-à-vis* the medical system, political activism among patients, and market-place competition and consumerism (Conrad and Leiter 2004; Mechanic 2002; Williams and Calnan 1996). But it also has to do with changes in the general medical world-view, i.e. how patients, bodies, diseases and treatments are perceived and considered.

The British medical sociologist David Armstrong has pointed out that at least from the early 1900s until the early 2000s medicine defined the body primarily through its three-dimensionality (Armstrong 2002). Diseases had their sites inside the body, in specific organs, structures and functions. For the medical doctor it was of great importance to be able to look into the body in order to be able to observe and understand lesions and pathologies. Basically this could be done in two ways. It could be done through the interpretation of signs and symptoms, or by using various techniques and instruments in order to *look* inside the body. Simple technological devices like the stethoscope and techniques like palpation made it possible to listen to the sounds of the body, and try to make an image of the functionality and structural aspects of organs (Reiser 1978). Later on, X-ray technology gave the medical doctor an opportunity to make *photos* of the inside of the body and thus be able to actually look into the body without opening it (Kevles 1997; Pasveer 1989; Reiser 1978).

Armstrong points out that during the early twentieth century medicine started to establish *functional* relationships between organs, their structures and functions, the ill person, and even later on, lifestyle. Pathologies were no longer just identified in structural deficiencies and pathologies of the organs inside the body, but in the functional relationship between the patient and his/her surroundings. Good examples of this are the relationship between smoking and cancer, or stress and cardiac infarction. This means that it is important for the doctor to get information from the patient not only about symptoms, but also about lifestyle factors in order to be able to establish a diagnosis and suggest a treatment regime.

It was not only the changes in the perception of bodies and diseases that affected the relationship between medical doctors and patients. Forces *outside* or *around* the medical institution have also affected the doctor–patient relationship. Medicine is still in many ways powerful in relation to patients. At the same time many chronically ill patients and their relatives have become organized in various support groups or patient organizations. In some instances there is strong support for the empowerment of patients in order to strengthen their rights and options in relation to the medical establishment (see for instance Gabe *et al.* 1994).

Many patients also have access to the Internet, which means that they can search for information about their specific conditions, their treatments and prognoses. This makes it possible to compare the information provided by the doctor with information gathered on the Internet. In this way patients become increasingly able to challenge and negotiate even the terms of their own medical problems (Broom 2005; Nettleton *et al.* 2005; Radin 2006). Added to this is the increase in the use of complementary and alternative medicine (CAM) in the Western world (Eisenberg *et al.* 1998), which also challenges the traditional concentration of medical knowledge in the hands of the biomedical professionals and institutions. Furthermore, through changes in the financing and organization of the health care system, more patients have the option of choosing their own health care providers. On the other hand, it increases the influence of both private and national health insurance over the kind of medical care offered to patients.

As a consequence the ideals and norms for communication between doctor and patient have changed from being doctor-centred to being patient-centred. This was partly an effect of a changing medical world-view. Earlier communicative ideals stressed that the medical doctor should in principle be quite critical about what the patient says and base his/her medical diagnosis on signs rather than on the patient's account of symptoms. In order to achieve knowledge about how the patient functions in his/her life situation and hence be able to understand *functional* problems, the doctor had to pay more attention to the patient's symptoms; this was also important in order to increase compliance with treatment regimes.

All these changes in medicine affect the communicative patterns and the relationship between doctor and patient in the general area of negotiation and dialogue. The changes have resulted in the development of new *communicative technologies* and *ideologies* – technologies that do not basically differ from other medical technologies in that they mediate the relationship between doctor and patient.

One way of understanding the new communicative technologies and ideologies is to investigate how these are learnt. Surprisingly few studies have focused on the way medical students learn how to talk with patients – and most studies are concerned with comparing content and educational practices of communication skills training (Hargie *et al.* 1998), evaluating courses' effects (Aspegren 1999; Hulsman *et al.* 1999), or identifying background factors that enhance or hinder communicative performance (Suzuki Laidlaw *et al.* 2006) or effects on communication skills (Harms *et al.* 2004).

Medical programmes in communication are interesting because many of the phenomena that are integrated in daily medical practice and hence are taken for granted are the objects of deliberation and learning during medical education. Strategies, assumptions, norms and conventions that are part of the everyday medical communicative practice must be made explicit during the learning process in order for students to be able to understand and learn to organize their own communicative practices. Hence they become visible and possible to study and discuss.

Communicative ideologies and technologies

As we discussed above, the changes in medicine have gone from a one-sided perspective on the inner body to an interest in a functional perspective of the patient in his/her life-world context, resulting in an increased need for knowledge about the patient outside the clinic. Many other factors have also affected the relationship between medical doctor and patient. Most of these factors have to do with the social conditions and constraints of the health care system, like diminishing medical authority, emergence of medical shopping and patient activism. Through these developments new communicative needs emerge in the health care sector in general, and more specifically between doctors and patients.

Due to the development of medical technology a number of new communicative situations have emerged. This is especially true in areas where decisions have to made and the patient has to be involved, for instance in genetic counselling or when medical doctors or registered nurses have to try to get the patient to make a change in lifestyle (cf. Adelswärd and Sachs 1996, 1998; Sarangi 2000; Sarangi and Clarke 2002). In most of these areas the medical tasks are related to moral questions that involve the patient's life world and most often also relatives' lives.

These new communicative needs have resulted in the emergence of new *communicative technologies* and *ideologies*, that is, new ways and norms for how doctors should communicate with patients. This development is not unique to medicine; it can be seen in many other areas as well, for instance in the educational system and above all in the commercial market sector (see e.g. Cameron 2000; Fairclough 1992; Hochschild 1983).

Communicative technologies can be defined as 'transcontextual   techniques, which are seen as resources or tool-kits that can be used to pursue a wide variety of strategies in many diverse contexts' (Fairclough 1992: 215). Communicative ideologies have to do with the social and cultural norms that guide and provide information, for instance for conversations, and also serve as evaluative standards to show both good and bad examples of conversations. What Norman Fairclough calls *democratization of discourse*, defined as the removal of elements like discursive markers of inequality and power and the informalization of language use, is an example of a new communicative norm and ideology. The development of new communicative technologies and ideologies results not only in new linguistic and pragmatic norms, but also in new terminology and ways of talking about communication (cf. Cameron 2000).

Learning to communicate professionally often means learning how to use communicative technologies and the corresponding ideologies. Historically, professionals learned to talk with patients and clients by learning from senior colleagues (cf. Atkinson 1989), i.e. through a process of informal hands-off practical skills and experience. This is of course still the case, but communication has also become a topic of special educational programmes, and as a consequence learning to become a professional often also means learning specific communicative techniques. That is, the process of learning to talk with patients has become formalized.

In medicine these new communicative technologies and ideologies have been developed over recent decades, beginning in the 1970s (cf. the discussion in Armstrong 2002: 159–73, and the historical discussion in Atkinson 1989 and Hydén and Mishler 1999). Of central importance has been the idea that the medical doctor should not primarily talk *to* the patient, but rather *with* him/her. That is, the doctor should not only deliver the results of examinations and decisions about treatment but also discuss these results jointly with the patient in a *dialogue* format (Sarangi 2000). It is rather the dialogue than the one-sided delivery of information that stands out as a central, valued norm for communication with the patient. It is also important for the doctor to take into account and understand the patient's life world – or at least parts of it – in order to be able to interpret not only symptoms and signs but also to be able to suggest treatments that actually fit into the life situation of the patient (Kleinman 1988; Clark and Mishler 1992).

As almost all doctors run on tight time schedules it has become important to develop more or less specific communicative skills and strategies that make it possible for doctors to routinize their medical interviews. It must be possible to perform the medical interview in almost the same way irrespective of the actual patient, the type of medical problem, the specific situation or context – but also irrespective of the specific medical doctor. The medical interview still has to be performed in a way that lives up to the basic norms of communication and good doctoring. In other words, the communicative technology has to be independent of actual persons and their problems and conditions, and rather be a part of the health care organization.

Communication programme

During the past decade or so we have seen the emergence of more or less institutionalized educational measures in, for instance, the training of medical doctors in communicating with patients. Becoming a medical doctor not only involves learning the traditional biomedical knowledge, but also learning how to talk and interact with patients, how to evaluate this talk and how to talk about talk. That is, becoming a doctor also means learning how to observe, analyse and discuss one's own ways with patients as well as those of colleagues and students; i.e. learning to implement and use a communicative ideology. It is a self-reflective mode that has at least to some extent become part of the modern medical identity and competence.

This is not a trivial task for students, at least not in an academic setting, as most medical subjects are embedded in a system of academic medical specialities that can be mastered mainly by mere cognitive learning. Courses in medical communication therefore often contain practical elements that lead to an increased effect on communication skills. Yet, most efforts to optimize courses in doctor–patient communication focus on creating effective training modes, e.g. longitudinal versus concentrated instruction (van Dalen *et al.* 2002) and evaluation formats (Humphris and Kaney 2000; Humphris 2001). The assessment of students' acquired communication skills is regarded as a powerful motivational learning source.

As the acquisition of *professional* communication competence involves processes that differ from most traditional academic subjects, the special difficulties and requirements of such courses need to be highlighted and understood. Few studies of this process focus on the wider social context, and address the wider functions and meanings of doctor–patient communication. Most studies of communication in medical settings have focused on the ways doctors and patients talk together, and generally on the social and verbal interactive patterns and how these are structured by the institutional context. This is especially true of most studies in the conversation analytic tradition (see for instance Erickson 1999). Most of these studies do not discuss the communication processes in terms of technologies and communicative ideologies.

The Faculty of Health Sciences at Linköping University (Sweden) has given a course in communications skills training since 1986. It gives medical students from the first to the fourth academic term the opportunity to meet patients at a primary health care centre and to practise diagnostic interviews that focus on both the medical and the psychosocial aspects of the patient's illness. These interviews are recorded on videotapes and discussed in small groups together with a general practitioner and a group supervisor. Supervision groups usually consist of seven students, one general practitioner who is employed at the respective primary health care centre, and one group supervisor, often a therapist trained in group or family therapy. The student belongs to the same group throughout the course.

We followed two groups in Terms 1, 2 and 3 of the medical programme. The first group consisted of four female and three male students, and a male group supervisor; as the general practitioners changed during the course, two male and one female physician were in this group. The second group consisted of five female and two male students, one group supervisor and one general practitioner, both females.

The groups held their sessions at two different primary health care centres in two different Swedish towns. The sessions took place during the course of an afternoon and started with two students meeting one patient, one student talking and one videoing the interview. After the student–patient interview, both students sat in on the patient's regular visit to the general practitioner. The following group discussions included the collective watching of the filmed student–patient interviews accompanied by comments. Discussions were videoed.

Ideology and reflexivity

The medical communication taught at the Faculty of Health Sciences at Linköping University employs a communicative *ideology* that is based on a biopsychosocial perspective on health and illness and uses the physician's emotional perceptions of the patient as a diagnostic source. The course plan formulates educational objectives for each academic term. This involves confronting the student with increasingly difficult interview situations concerning disease severity and the patient's social background (age, ethnic group, foreign language). As a theoretical introduction, a book on the communication model is read, and there are guidelines for the skills to be acquired during the course. These guidelines are based on the biopsychosocial model and ideology and operationalize its assumptions in the doctor–patient relationship.

A *holistic* perspective on the communication model takes the patient's life situation as well as his/her psychosocial background and current relationships into account. The model is viewed in the training programme as presenting a *patient-centred* point of view in contrast to a *disease-centred* or *doctor-centred* one. Physicians using a patient-centred approach to history-taking in the sense characterized above are supposed to actively help their patients to talk about their life situation and take into account the patients' diagnostic ideas. The conversational style includes what is called an *open attitude* that aims at *encountering the patient as a person*, to get into close contact and a *dialogue* by listening to his/her story. Such an approach implies also that the students learn to abandon a certain degree of control over the conversation and hand it over to the patients, to practise *an emotional, empathetic attitude*, and to be sensitive to non-verbal signs.

After having completed the course in communication skills during the fourth academic term, students undergo an examination where they meet a patient and take a medical history. The interview is also evaluated according to the students' communicative behaviour, focusing on the main features of the response model as summarized in an examination sheet. On this form, nine communicative abilities are specified and described in detail, making a systematic evaluation possible. This kind of evaluation form is used at different universities and has proved to indicate performance well and to be positively correlated to training (Humphris 2001).

Learning new routinized techniques that are going to be used in various medical contexts for performing different types of tasks also means learning to talk about talk. It means, for instance, interpreting different types of communicative situations, identifying communicative problems and finding solutions to these problems and evaluating instances of doctor–patient communication in terms of good and bad examples. It means especially learning how to talk with colleagues about talk – both one's own talk and theirs.

The students studied here learned to talk about talk in their group sessions together with their supervisors and senior colleagues. The discussions had a case- and problem-focusing structure that centred on the encounter between the student and the patient. The discussions aimed at analysing the particular student's strengths and weaknesses in communicating in a *professional* way and at discussing these on a general level that concerned the whole student group. Both the improvement of individual expertise and a heightened consciousness for problematic interview situations were strived for.

The student's account of the interview served as a starting point for the group discussions. The student who met the patient opened with a short case presentation, complemented by his/her impressions of the interview and a tentative analysis of shortcomings that he/she experienced with regard to the communication. Sometimes the student expressed some precise problems that he/she experienced and for which he/she requested help from the group. This phase took at most five minutes.

The video was then turned on and watched by the group, sometimes after each student had been assigned an aspect to which he/she was to pay certain attention, e.g. how the student formulated questions, or how he/she used body language.

One group member, often the supervisor or the student who conducted the interview, then stopped the tape at a point that they thought illustrated the initially formulated problem, or some other critical aspect of the interview situation. Then discussion started and often focused on two aspects. First the student's problem had to be identified and formulated into a learning need, and secondly some form of remedial action had to be suggested. These two foci formed the basis of the group discussion.

Interaction problems discussed in the groups

A wide range of recurring problem areas connected with interviewing patients in a *professional* way was discussed in the groups. The identification of the problem and the specification of an appropriate remedial action were embedded in a dynamic process that recurred on several sources – the videotape, the student's perceptions, and impressions by other group members – and were interwoven with the discussion of possible solutions. It was common for several problems from different *areas* to be formulated in the course of the discussion, before they were discussed in an exhaustive way and before solutions were found. Some problems remained unanswered or were reacted to with a long time delay.

The degree of active involvement by the peer group and the supervisors also varied with the kind of problem, and the discussion level oscillated between the student's own difficulties and general reflections about the topic.

Basically three different types of problems tended to recur in the discussions. The first type was problems related to communicative *skills*, like being able to organize and lead the interview, keep to the agenda, and so on. The second type of problem had to do with the *transformation of identity*, that is, learning to differentiate between the private and personal on the one hand and the professional on the other hand. This includes learning to see both oneself and the patient within the framework of a professional relationship. It also includes learning *self-reflection*; i.e. how to talk about talk in a group of colleagues.

The communicative technologies used in medical practice as well as in other settings all take everyday talk and communicative practices as their – often implicit – foundation. Learning to develop new ways of talking with patients is then basically about using everyday practices in new ways (see the discussion in Drew and Heritage 1992).

In everyday talk, both parties contribute to and negotiate the situation of what they are doing, what they are talking about, etc. Talk between doctor and patient, on the other hand, is defined by institutional and professional norms and constraints, tasks and goals, and imposes certain expectations and roles on both doctor and patient. In everyday talk, the interaction between the participants is negotiated and in most cases turns are fairly even distributed in terms of who talks the most or who decides what to talk about. In the doctor/patient talk, it is the doctor who sets the agenda, who conducts the interview and decides when and what to talk about. That is, asymmetric relations in the medical professional context replace the more or less symmetrical relations between participants in everyday conversations (cf. Drew and Heritage 1992; Sarangi and Roberts 1999).

This means that medical students have to learn to interact in new ways in the medical interview situation. The symmetrical relation has to be developed into an asymmetrical one. This is not a simple cognitive task of just learning to think and act differently; rather it involves a changed self- and role-perception on the part of the medical student. As a consequence it also means developing a new kind of relationship to persons as patients. It also implies learning to *violate* certain fundamental interactional rules. Instances of this rule violation include not telling a story about your own medical problems in response to the patient telling his/her story, or being able to interrupt patients in order to get specific kinds of answers to your questions, or being able to ask about sensitive topics, like family life or sexual matters.

If some everyday practices are violated others are *overemphasized*. This may include being very careful about the opening and the closing of the encounter in order to give the patients or clients the opportunity to express their concerns and questions and check if they want to bring up something more. Being aware of and using non-verbal communicative resources is another example. This includes everything from the way the physical setting is organized and how the participants face each other, to the way eye contact and intonation are handled (see Heath 1986; Hydén and Baggens 2004).

Some of the problems that surfaced in the group discussion had to do with the fact that the medical students had to redefine their relationships with other persons in the medical context – especially with patients, but also with other types of medical professionals. They are no longer just one person meeting another person, being able to talk about things like physical problems, but rather a medical doctor encountering a patient who expects and demands professional help. Learning to become a medical doctor involves changing situational definition and interactional format in talk.

Finally, a central aspect of learning to communicate professionally is developing a professional *identity* that is reflexive and is different from one's private identity. This is accomplished in many ways (cf. the classical study by Becker *et al.* 1961/1977), but most importantly through the way talk is organized (Hydén 2000). Learning, for instance, to distinguish between the professional and personal voice, and listening to and interacting with patients not as fellow human beings but as patients, means developing a new professional identity. Learning modern communicative techniques also means learning to be self-reflective about interaction and language use, and developing skills for discussing these issues with other colleagues. In other words, the identity that is developed not only has the classical attributes of professional identity but is also, most importantly, self-reflective.

In the following we give some examples from the group discussions.

Skills: organizing the interview

One important technique that the students had to learn to use is how to structure the medical interview with the help of the communicative model used in their training. This ideological model of medical communication sketches the main traits of successful doctor–patient communication, both in temporal form and interview content.

Some students had problems with internalizing and realizing these guidelines, or did not know how to apply them to a concrete case. Where does the patient's presentation of his or her complaint start and end, when is it time to become directive and where is the right place for a summary? What does the understanding of one's own and the patient's reactions mean, and what signifies professional empathy?

These are common questions that confront medical students, especially in the beginning of their experience with patient contact. Some students did not agree with the model and felt a need to discuss it critically. Also, the general practitioner's and the group supervisor's conduct in encountering patients, sometimes served as a more vivid impression of *good* patient–physician communication as compared with the formal model by which the students were supposed to be guided. In general the students identified a need to reflect upon the model and find their personal styles of adopting it.

Stopping the videotape, one student wondered how she could encourage the patient to give a complete account of his complaints before she summarizes the interview:

Example 1a

STUDENT: I could not get it out (...) after having asked him several times if
    he had any other complaints I was ready to summarize the interview just
    when I tried to summarize he said:
    'Yeah, last year in September I had an operation for prostate tumour'
    you know
    then he started coming up with [more problems]
    how might one try to encourage patients to mention their complaints
    and symptoms before one summarizes?

Other common difficulties concerned with the interview's structure were how to plan an optimal time disposal, how to control the length of a patient's account, the best point of time for initiating a new interview phase and how to handle situations in which the patient did not follow the agenda.

Many students had difficulties in establishing a mutually open relationship with the patient. Some felt unable to adopt a therapeutic attitude towards the patient, while others felt unable to locate a specific problem in the particular patient's report about symptoms and ailments.

In general, problems with the relationship between physician and patient often constituted the backbone of the discussions, and were modified from a general to a specific level, i.e. from a general feeling to instances of 'true' interactive behaviour.

Help from the group included a detailed analysis of the interaction, i.e. finding some hints in the video about whether the problem was in the student's or the patient's behaviour. The general practitioner's professional experience was often demanded, and practical suggestions for handling similar kinds of situations or patients were sought. In some cases the student's overall attitude towards patient–physician relations had to be considered.

Typical complaints concerning the doctor–patient relationship included having problems with defining the professional role (in degree of authority, display of trustworthiness, etc.), being able to establish a good contact – i.e. avoiding a failed sense of rapport or compatibility with the patient – and achieving a *balanced* verbal activity by not dominating the interview too much.

This student is not satisfied with the interview's general *flow* as he does not perceive a balanced activity and a feeling of establishing a *dialogue*. He ascribes this primarily to his own stressed and insecure mental attitude (Example 1b).

Example 1b

STUDENT: Well I just think
  I can't get a conversation going
  It's like
  It's not relax-
  or rather I'm not relaxed
  and then
  like
  then I become stressed just by asking
  and then I can't figure out what to say
  I was not sure when I was sitting there
  just like that
  well
  I didn't feel secure
  It was difficult to get him to feel secure and start telling me.

In Example 2 a student in the group discussions reflects upon the communicative characteristics that are ascribed to a doctor by virtue of his professional role and status.

Example 2

STUDENT: We are medical students
  we don't look like doctors
  I mean

if one had a white coat
one would adopt the doctor's role much more obviously.
SUPERVISOR: Kind of more authority …
STUDENT: No
that one acts more as a professional than as a fellow human being
rather because with a doctor one can talk quite frankly from the
beginning
one can talk with a different trust the first time one meets them.

This student apparently draws on the communicative ideology and models of professional doctoring as being about virtues like frankness and trust, in contrast to the moral and psychological properties of ordinary men.

Identity transformation

Learning to talk professionally is not only about learning certain skills, but also about changed self-perception, or rather, a transformation of identity. Learning to talk professionally is learning to talk *as if* one is a certain kind of professional person, in this case a medical doctor. The voice has to become that of a doctor. But it is also necessary to learn to perceive the patient and what he or she says in terms of a patient speaking to (or with) a doctor. That is, it is not only learning to speak that is central to the identity transformation, but also learning to interpret the action of the patient in professional terms, and then respond as a professional.

In order to talk professionally it is important for the students to be able to detach the actual voices used in the medical interview from their private voices (Example 3).

Example 3

STUDENT: You have to be able to say to a patient
    'What a pity!'
    and sound convincing, but if he [the patient] says
    'I'll probably have to become a disability pensioner'
    then I will have trouble saying 'What a pity!' convincingly.

Learning to use *empathy* as an interactive instrument is perceived as especially difficult by many students. The reason for this is probably that it includes a mental attitude that most of the students usually display towards close friends or other people with whom they have personal relationships. Adopting a professional identity that includes *empathic feedback* towards persons with whom they are otherwise unacquainted has to be tested and integrated in their own ways of speaking and being.

Example 4

STUDENT: Even if I can understand
  it feels like I'm
  I have problems with professional empathy because I can recognize it
  but it's not me
  genuinely
  but it is
  I know I should reassure the patient, but when I confirm that I actually
  understood I don't have the genuine feeling.

Learning to communicate as a doctor also means using language in a professional way, i.e. conducting certain interactive (speech) actions, such as formulating questions that aim at eliciting the patient's report, directing the patient's account, and giving a certain kind of feedback.

In the group discussions one specific type of speech action seemed to cause special trouble, specifically that of asking questions. The students have to learn about formulating questions, but also to put their questions in the correct (medical) order, such as exploring the major bodily systems in a certain order.

Example 5

STUDENT (commenting on another student):
  I think the contents of the questions were okay
  although the questions were a bit circumscribed
  you said: 'You have not ...'
  but the order of your questions was okay I think
  it was logical.

Instead, an open invitation is suggested for the patient's account, and the students are trained to become increasingly sensitive to identifying phrases that help the patient to talk openly about his/her life situation.

Example 6

STUDENT: Just repeat what the patient just said
  'Oh you play golf!'
  and then you go quiet [laughter in the group].
SUPERVISOR: I think it's good to do it like that
  because you also connect to the patient
  maybe you talk about other things for a while
  but it's okay
  let the ends justify the means as long as it brings you forward and you
  can establish a relationship.

Another area is learning to talk about and specifically ask questions about sensitive topics like family life, economic situation, mental health or sexuality. One aim of the course is to encourage the students to adopt a holistic approach to medical interviewing, which means considering the interplay of the patient's body, psyche, ethnicity, and environment in different life contexts. This perspective demands the exploration of the patient's social background, his/her family, occupation, and his/her own reflections about his/her physical condition. Yet many students do not know how they can address such private aspects of the patient's life in an appropriate way, or feel that they cannot justify their curiosity about the patient's life. Some students are afraid to be confronted with emotional accounts that they cannot handle.

Students often requested help from the group with legitimizing the intrusion into the patient's privacy, and also with ways of expressing interest in the patient's life circumstances.

Example 7

STUDENT: It is just as hard for us to talk about mental problems as it is for them
and it is much easier not to dig around in it because these are quite intricate questions addressing 'stress' and asking questions like
'Do you feel depressed?'
I think it's easier to talk about one's shoulder than asking
'Are you anxious?'
but this it what we have to learn.

Sensitive topics are those that students perceive as hard to address and that they assume the patients would find it hard to talk about. The main problem for students in this situation is their own emotional reaction to, and the resulting responsibility for the patient's emotional well-being. Talking about physical complaints and those aspects of the patient's lifestyle that are related to physical behaviour (eating, smoking, sports, etc.) is nowadays no longer perceived as difficult. Instead, asking about a person's family and issues like separation and related problems around child custody, or lack of friends and social support is not easy for most students, especially if the direct relevance to the medical diagnosis is not apparent at first glance. As the interview model taught in the course and the patient-centred attitude demand an interest in the patient's life, the students on the other hand feel pressured to touch on those subjects.

Learning self-reflection

In the group discussions students and supervisors all made contributions to the discussion in response to some kind of perceived problem. The suggestions they came up with were related to and shaped by the kinds of difficulties with interviewing patients that are taken up by students, and are thus individually tailored. Like what was said about problems, the suggestions appeared during different discussion parts, and were frequently interrupted by other activities, such as watching the videotape and formulating problems. The suggestions were expressed at different levels of specificity, were modified during the discussion, and were given from a variety of perspectives – the students' view, the GP's professional experience, and the group supervisor's perspective.

In general, the suggestions were aimed at mediating and elaborating on the response model presented above, and at deepening an understanding of its practical implications. They not only had the function of solving actual problems, but also of providing the students with cognitive resources, i.e. a terminology for describing, analysing and structuring professional medical talk and interaction.

Discussing the videoed student–patient encounters has the function of increasing the student's awareness of the structure of medical interviews and its typical interactive elements. In a general comment during a group discussion a supervisor summarizes the general communicative ideology and its functions:

Example 8

SUPERVISOR: This course is about giving you the chance to learn to get to
    know yourself in this situation
    encountering the patient
    the way you usually act and react
    what you feel
    what you do
    what your strong and weak sides are.
    And maybe it is about starting to understand something
    'Well sometimes I need to take a break because otherwise I will ask two
    questions at the same time and then I get rather lost'
    or whatever
    the important thing to learn during this course is finding your own
    style
    the way you work.

Being aware of one's communicative behaviour and monitoring the interview's process requires an increased cognitive effort. A useful aid for doctors-to-be is a repertoire of procedural heuristics for recognizing and handling typical interview situations. Such procedural knowledge concerning the physician's thoughts and reflections-in-action (Schön 1983) is mainly extracted from the general practitioner's and the group supervisor's professional experience. An important aspect is also the patient's assumed perspective and how it can be brought into the physician's actions. Solutions that aim at providing heuristic advice for typical interview situations are often formulated on a general level.

The advice given typically covered areas like learning to recognize the emotional value and tone of a patient's account, knowing the appropriate point of time for interactive actions (for instance when and how to react to emotionally loaded accounts and giving feedback to the patient) and learning to differentiate between relevant and less relevant information. The advice could also cover learning to use metaphoric expressions in interviews (for instance forming a *picture* or a *jigsaw puzzle* of the patient's life) and interpreting hints from the patient that could signal a hidden problem.

Example 9

SUPERVISOR: Hm okay,
      we don't need to make such a big thing out of it
      but I think that this is something to think about.
      When one meets a patient who so apparently sends signals about
      something painful and troublesome,
      that we in one way or another have to respond to that.

Another recurrent area of advice concerned how to manage the interaction in the medical interview. Much of this advice had to do with learning how to be in command in the interview situation.

Example 10

SUPERVISOR: So maybe it is good to give oneself a bit of time in order to
      think and formulate the question
      not to be in a hurry
      let it become a bit quiet
      be calm
      see if you like
      can think about the information you got.

Even if an interview situation can get stuck, acting in a professional way means improvising and using a doctor's full communicative repertoire in order to *get all* the necessary diagnostic information. This GP suggests – in a slightly jocular manner – a combination of verbal interaction with physical examination, for instance. He encourages the students to take their time to reflect and actively change the process of an interview, instead of judging their actions in terms of *right* or *wrong*.

Example 11

DOCTOR: I think it is important to find some time for reflection
   if you don't feel comfortable then as a doctor you can always do
   something else in the meantime [laughs]
   you can take an EKG
   or fake a phone call [laughs]
   no but seriously
   sometimes you have to take time out and think
   'What the hell, I'll have to start all over again'
   or at least start on a new track.

Another piece of advice given to the student is to develop and use patient typologies. According to the supervisors, meeting each patient's special communicative needs becomes easier when patients are classified and categorized. These categories can be based on the patient's social characteristics, such as age, gender, and profession, or on his/her disease, or his/her attitude towards health care, which includes the patient's expectations of the encounter. Typologies offer simplifications that can serve as cognitive support in future encounters and are sometimes provided by the GP or the group supervisor or elaborated on during the discussion. One example of categories used is young patients versus old patients.

Example 12

DOCTOR: Well a vigorous patient born in the 1920s doesn't visit a doctor
   until he has multiple symptoms.
   Do you see what I'm saying?
STUDENT: Isn't that very sound?
   You only visit the doctor when
DOCTOR: Sound to visit a doctor!
   But that's dangerous!
   [laughs]
DOCTOR: Yeah I mean
   People in the generation born in the 1920s when there weren't that
   many doctors around generally don't visit the doctor once every three
   months
   so when they do, I interpret it as the person's really being worried.

Other recurrent categories are academically educated patients versus uneducated patients, physically ill patients versus psychosomatically ill patients or mentally ill patients, and acute versus chronically ill patients. Some of the categories pertain to psychological characteristics, or have to do with being a reserved or silent patient versus being a communicative and talkative patient.

Example 13

SUPERVISOR: Is this patient a sensitive person
     or is he like a computer
     or whatever you want to call him?
     When he tells you about his problems
     which of these labels do you think works for you?

Students often demanded concrete help in coping with difficult interview situations in a professional way. Adopting standard formulations helps them to feel more confident in their new roles. Professional expressions and standard meanings were mainly obtained from the general practitioner's and the group supervisor's stock of experience, but fellow students can also contribute helpful comments. In particular, sensitive topics and their unfamiliar levels of intimacy are more easily mastered with the help of *approved* phrases that are sometimes tested in short role-plays. Often this does not mean formulation of intricate questions but rather opening the field for the patient's thoughts and experiences in a *confidential* and *safe* way.

Typical areas that can be mastered with the help of professional formulations include posing open, exploratory questions, being directive in a polite and professional way (e.g. interrupting a talkative patient) or addressing sensitive topics.

Finally, the students are encouraged to use their personal experience in talking with persons they meet for the first time. The use of everyday talk in order to establish an atmosphere of trust is explicitly approved.

Discussion and concluding remarks

In his book *A New History of Identity* (2002) David Armstrong makes the remark that 'the transformative process whereby the student was made into a professional could be made transparent, no longer shrouded in initiation mysteries' (2002: 175). What medical students learn in learning to communicate with patients is how to use certain everyday practices in order to be able to pursue their professional goals and tasks most effectively.

Communication skills and strategies have become integrated parts of modern medical practice and the way the medical organization works. Learning to communicate in this sense has less to do with listening to the voice of the patient and more to do with learning a technology that serves the medical practice and organization. David Mechanic expresses this quite well when he writes:

> We can (...) develop organizational systems that help people behave like good people and avoid incentives and systems that result in adverse events.
>
> (Mechanic 2002)

Talking about professional medical talk and especially one's own communicative style in the professional role requires a certain awareness of language and interaction that most students do not possess from the beginning, but which they acquire during the group discussions.

Classifying one's own interactive actions as an affective response or as interrupting the patient's story and taking responsibility for the interview's progress, time schedule and talk in a self-monitoring way – these are the skills that are acquired from training and reflection. The group setting and the discussion allow the adoption and development of a common *language* to describe communicative processes and to apply it to oneself – and this may be the main difference between this situation and mere individual bedside training and unreflected professional experience.

Above all, learning to talk and interact with patients in modern medicine involves learning to be self-reflective and being able to reflect together with colleagues. This includes being able to look at video recordings of one's own and others' interactions with patients, and being able to analyse, discuss and contribute suggestions and helpful reflections in a discussion. Through this process a representation of a prescribed style of doctoring and of being a doctor is presented, learned and reproduced. Armstrong writes that it is 'the creation of a doctor, by a doctor, for view by other doctors' (2002: 169). The doctor becomes a true professional in the eye of the other doctor – less so in the eye of the patient.

Acknowledgment

Antje Lumma's work on this chapter has been supported by a grant from the Swedish Research Council.

References

Adelswärd, V. and Sachs, L. (1996) 'A nurse in preventive work: dilemmas of health information talks', *Scandinavian Journal of Caring Science*, 10: 45–52.

Adelswärd, V. and Sachs, L. (1998) 'Risk discourse: recontextualization of numerical values in clinical practice', *Text*, 18: 191–210.

Armstrong, D. (2002) *A New History of Identity: A Sociology of Medical Knowledge*, London: Palgrave.

Aspegren, K. (1999) 'BEME Guide No. 2: teaching and learning communication skills in medicine – a review with quality grading of articles', *Medical Teacher*, 21: 563–70.

Atkinson, P. (1989) 'Review essay: Voices from the past: a historical note on the discourse of medical instruction', *Sociology of Health and Illness*, 11: 78–82.

Becker, H.S., Geer, B., Hughes, E.C. and Strauss, A.L. (1977) *Boys in White: Student Culture in Medical School*, New Brunswick, NJ: Transaction Publishers.

Broom, A. (2005) 'Virtually He@lthy: the impact of internet use on disease experience and the doctor–patient relationship', *Qualitative Health Research*, 15: 325–45.

Cameron, D. (2000) *Good to Talk?*, London: Sage.

Clark, J.A. and Mishler, E.G. (1992) 'Attending patient's stories: reframing the clinical task', *Sociology of Health and Illness*, 14: 344–71.

Conrad, P. (2005) 'The shifting engines of medicalization', *Journal of Health and Social Behavior*, 46: 3–14.

Conrad, P. and Leiter, V. (2004) 'Medicalization, markets and consumers', *Journal of Health and Social Behavior*, 45 (Extra issue): 158–76.

Drew, P. and Heritage, J. (1992) 'Analyzing talk at work: an introduction', in P. Drew and J. Heritage (eds) *Talk At Work: Interaction in Institutional Settings*, Cambridge: Cambridge University Press.

Eisenberg, D., Davis, R., Ettner, S., Appel, L.S., Wilkey, S. and Van Rompay, M. (1998) 'Trends in alternative medicine use in the United States, 1990–1997: results of a follow-up national survey', *Journal of the American Medical Association*, 280: 1569–75.

Erickson, F. (1999) 'Appropriation of voice and presentation of self as a fellow physician: aspects of discourse of apprenticeship in medicine', in S. Sarangi and C. Roberts (eds) *Talk, Work and Institutional Order: Discourse in Medical, Mediation and Management Settings*, Berlin: Mouton de Gruyter.

Fairclough, N. (1992) *Discourse and Social Change*, Cambridge: Polity Press.

Gabe, J., Kelleher, D. and Williams G. (eds) (1994) *Challenging Medicine*, London: Routledge.

Hargie, O., Dickson, D., Boohan, M. and Hughes, K. (1998) 'A survey of communication skills training in UK Schools of Medicine: present practices and prospective proposals', *Medical Education*, 32: 25–34.

Harms, C. Y., Jr, Amsler, F., Zettler, C., Scheidegger, D. and Kindler, C. H. (2004) 'Special article: improving anaesthetists' communication skills', *Anaesthesia*, 59: 166–72.

Heath, C. (1986) *Body Movement and Speech in Medical Interaction*, Cambridge: Cambridge University Press.

Hochschild, A.R. (1983) *The Managed Heart: Commercialization of Human Feeling*, Berkeley: University of California Press.

Hulsman, R.L., Winnubst, J.A. and Bensing, J.M. (1999) 'Teaching clinical experienced physicians communication skills: a review of evaluation studies', *Medical Education*, 33: 655–68.

Humphris, G.M. and Kaney, S. (2000) 'The objective structured video exam for assessment of communication skills', *Medical Education*, 34: 939–45.

Humphris, G.M.K. (2001) 'The Liverpool brief assessment system for communication skills in the making of doctors', *Advances in Health Sciences Education*, 6: 69–80.

Hydén, L.C. (2001) 'Who!? Identity in institutional contexts', in M. Seltzer, C. Kullberg, S.P. Olesen and I. Rostila (eds), *Listening to the Welfare State*, Aldershot: Ashgate.

Hydén, L.C. and Baggens, C. (2004) 'Joint working relationships: children, parents and child healthcare nurses at work', *Communication and Medicine*, 1: 71–83.

Hydén, L.C. and Mishler, E.G. (1999) 'Medicine and language', *Annual Review of Applied Linguistics*, 19: 174–92.

Kevles, B.H. (1997) *Naked to the Bone: Medical Imagining in the Twentieth Century*, New Brunswick, NJ: Rutgers University Press.

Kleinman, A. (1988) *The Illness Narratives: Suffering, Healing, and the Human Condition*, New York: Basic Books.

Mechanic, D. (2002) 'Socio-cultural implications of changing organizational technologies in the provision of care', *Social Science and Medicine*, 54: 459–67.

Nettleton, S., Burrows, R. and O'Malley, L. (2005) 'The mundane realities of the everyday lay use of the internet for health, and their consequences for media convergence', *Sociology of Health and Illness*, 27: 972–92.

Pasveer, B. (1989) 'Knowledge of shadows: the introduction of X-ray images in medicine', *Sociology of Health and Illness*, 11: 360–81.

Radin, P. (2006) '"To me, it's my life": Medical communication, trust, and activism in cyberspace', *Social Science and Medicine*, 62: 591–601.

Reiser, S.J. (1978) *Medicine and the Reign of Technology*, Cambridge: Cambridge University Press.

Sarangi, S. (2000) 'Activity types, discourse types and interactional hybridity: the case of genetic counselling', in S. Sarangi and M. Coulthard (eds) *Discourse and Social Life*, London: Longman.

Sarangi, S. and Clarke, A. (2002) 'Zones of expertise and the management of uncertainty in genetics risk communication', *Research on Language and Social Interaction*, 35: 139–71.

Sarangi, S. and Roberts, C. (eds) (1999) *Talk, Work and Institutional Order: Discourse in Medical, Mediation and Management Settings*, Berlin: Mouton de Gruyter.

Schön, D.A. (1983) *The Reflective Practitioner: How Professionals Think in Action*, New York: Basic Books.

Suzuki Laidlaw, T.K., MacLeod, H., van Zanten, S., Simpson, D. and Wrixon, W. (2006) 'Relationship of resident characteristics, attitudes, prior training and clinical knowledge to communication skills performance', *Medical Education*, 40: 18–25.

van Dalen, J., Kerkhofs, E., van Knippenberg-van den Berg, B.W., van den Hout, B.W., Scherpbier, H.A. and van der Vleuten, C.P. (2002) 'Longitudinal and concentrated communication skills programmes: two Dutch medical schools compared', *Advances in Health Sciences Education*, 7: 29–40.

Williams, S.J. and Calnan, M. (1996) 'The "limits" of medicalization?: modern medicine and the lay populace in "late" modernity', *Social Science and Medicine*, 42: 1609–20.

3 What's in a Pap smear?

Biology, culture, technology and self in the cytology laboratory

Anette Forss

Introduction

The Papanicolaou (Pap) smear, also called the Pap test, cyto test, cervical smear or cervical cytology, has been described as the most widely used and established cancer-screening technology in the world. It has also been described as a very simple technology including a brush, a microscope slide, fixative and cervical cells from women. In 1928, George N. Papanicolaou, a Medical Doctor, investigator, PhD in zoology and Aureli Babes (1928/1967), a Romanian pathologist, each independently claimed to have found a 'very simple' technique, which provided a new possibility for early diagnostics of cancer/malignant tumours in the female genital tract/uterine cervix. The technique was subsequently named after Papanicolaou who, according to Wied (1964: 174), was more successful than Babes in 'stimulating the introduction of mass screening projects which are the actual benefit of the method'.[1]

In Sweden and other countries the Pap smear technology triggered what is today an established secondary preventive intervention directed towards 'healthy' women to detect those at risk for developing cervical cancer, a potentially fatal disease, as well as those with the disease (Royal National Board of Health 1966). Today, approximately 950,000 Pap smear tests are carried out each year, within and outside organised screening in Sweden (Swedish National Board of Health and Welfare 1998).[2] Further testing and medical follow-up is needed in approximately 4 per cent of the cases (ibid.).

Approximately 260, mostly female, cytodiagnosticians examine the vast majority of Pap smears in Sweden. They have no direct contact with the women taking the Pap smears. Their daily work involves the visualisation and interpretation of small excerpts from living human bodies, an essential component in the larger context of cervical cancer screening. As the vast majority of the Pap smears are normal the identification of normal cells constitutes the bulk of a cytodiagnostician's work. The cytodiagnosticians expertise concerns cytology.[3] They distinguish between normal cells and cells showing pathological changes by examining cytology samples down the microscope, which involves interpreting and classifying cells along a continuum between normal and pathological cells (Posner 1993). There have been very few qualitative studies on the cytodiagnosticians' work with this technology (see Singleton's 1998 UK-based study and Morris *et al*. 2001). As pointed out by Casper and Clarke (1998), commonly used technologies that are supposedly simple are often under-studied.

In this chapter I will discuss how the cytodiagnosticians create meaning in their daily work of analysing and classifying cells, and how they use the microscope and visual knowledge in such work. I will draw on data from a one-year ethnographic study conducted at one public and one private clinical routine cytology laboratory in urban Sweden, documented by field notes and interviews, in which the personnel were followed in their daily work.[4]

The cytology laboratory as ethnographic field

Ethnographic and/or qualitative studies on personnel's work with cells in cytology laboratories are scarce. When mentioned in the literature, the cytology laboratory is mostly enmeshed in the cervical cancer screening 'success story' (Koss 1989, Singleton 1998a, 1998b) and thereby implicitly rendered as a site where truths are created. Symonds (1997: 276) claims that Sweden is one of the countries with successful 'well-organised screening programmes', which 'can substantially reduce cervical cancer deaths'. The cytology laboratory may however, in contrast, also be part of cervical cancer screening 'failure stories' (Koss 1989, Singleton 1998a, 1998b). For example, occasionally various forms of misconduct associated with this type of screening are revealed.[5]

When the cytology laboratory has been described as a part of the success or failure discourses of cervical cancer screening, the cytology laboratory personnel's work has been concealed rather than revealed. When part of a success story, the test and results are most often understood as solely the outcomes of a mechanical process. Here, the interactions between technology (the Pap smear procedures), scientific disciplines (cytology and public health), a laudable social goal and value (cancer prevention through population screening), and a practice (professionals using technology to interpret and classify human cells within the context of both cytology and screening aims) are overlooked. When part of a failure story, human beings are often understood as the weak link in an otherwise advanced system. The mistakes and misinterpretations are explained by 'the human factor'. The cytology laboratory personnel's understandings of their work remain unstudied.

Ethnographic studies have previously been performed in *scientific* laboratories (Lynch 1985, 1988; Latour and Woolgar 1986; Traweek 1988; Knorr Cetina and Amann 1990; Rabinow 1996) as well as in routine *clinical* laboratories (Rapp 1999; Mol 2000; Keating and Cambrosio 2000). Although the ways of describing and drawing conclusions on laboratory work and the objects analysed diverge, there seems to be a general agreement among social scientists that important knowledge is produced in laboratories. Knorr Cetina (2001: 8232) claims that the laboratory 'epitomizes modern science and knowledge'. In a postscript to the second edition of the pioneering book *Laboratory Life, the Construction of Scientific Facts* (Latour and Woolgar 1986), the sociologist Bruno Latour describes how he realised (while in the Ivory Coast as a researcher) that to divide and to discriminate between scientific knowledge and farmers' knowledge was problematic. He therefore decided to apply the same field methods used to study Ivory Coast farmers for studying first-rate scientists. Latour performed an ethnographic study on, as he describes, a 'tribe of scientists' and 'their production of science' (p. 17) at an endocrinology laboratory at the Salk Institute. The work here, writes Latour, 'is commonly heralded as having a startling or, at least, extremely significant effects on our civilisation' (p. 17). One major conclusion from Latour and Woolgar's study is that scientific activity should not be seen as rendering a mirror of nature; instead the laboratory is a place where reality is constructed.

The anthropologist Laura Nader (1972), though not speaking specifically about the laboratory, has in a similar vein emphasised the importance of studying the production of authoritative knowledge, and called upon researchers to 'ask "common sense" questions in reverse' (p. 289) in their 'own' societies. The studies on taken-for-granted authoritative knowledge and on scientists in one's own society as exemplified by Nader and Latour and Woolgar, have been a source of inspiration for me. The basic assumptions in my study, however, differ from Latour's, as I do not wish to emulate his defamiliarisation and 'exotisation' of the laboratory and laboratory scientists, e.g. by referring to them as a tribe. Furthermore, Latour's focus seems to be on the production of scientific knowledge, whereas his 'tribe of scientists', the specific producers, remain rather invisible.

Magnifying the invisible

Today we may take the cell, diagnostic classifications, and the technological means for magnifying and rendering cells visible for granted, as technologies of visualisation now have, as Birke (1999:76) says, 'become part of the social processes by which we come to understand what it means to "see" inside the body'. Cartwright (1995) reminds us to scrutinise the co-evolution of visualisation technologies and medical knowledge. Different forms of 'static' and 'moving' visual technologies are in fact intertwined with different fields of medical knowledge of the body's inside, she argues. For example, the cinema, 'a technology designed to record and reproduce movement' (ibid. xii), was practically and ideologically associated with physiology. In contrast:

the static medium of photography was regarded within nineteenth-century science, medicine and state institutions as an instrument particularly well suited to the study of anatomy and morphology.

(Cartwright 1995: xii)

As seen above, Cartwright relates morphology (form and structure) to a static visualisation technology: the photographic picture. In cytology laboratories cell morphology is interpreted with another visual technology: the microscope. It is important to consider that neither the microscope nor the cell simply 'is' in the realm of biomedicine and cancer disease prevention. Indeed, the term 'cell' seems to be intertwined with and dependent on the microscope. According to medical historians, the word 'cell' was first used in 1665 when the English scientist Robert Hooke put a piece of cork under a microscope and distinguished compartments which he called 'cells' (Singer and Underwood 1962: 132). At times, the microscope has been discussed simultaneously with the telescope (see e.g. Butler *et al.* 1986; Fox Keller 1996; McGrath 2002). Both instruments emerged during the first decade of the seventeenth century and both can be seen as mediators: the telescope revealing outer space and the microscope revealing small parts of nature and the human body.

McGrath (2002) discusses shifting communication problems in regard to the representation of what was seen in the microscope from the seventeenth until the nineteenth century. For example, 'in order to have currency, foreign objects had to be translated into imagery' (ibid.: 171). The early microscopists drew sketches: later they used photographs. Since 'the specimen did not speak for itself but had to be read' (ibid.: 164), there were difficulties in accounting for and recognising what was seen, especially for new phenomena which lacked material for comparison. To gain credibility for the claims of what was seen the use of mechanical standards and formal properties such as 'shape, colour, edge or border, size, transparency, surface' were emphasised.[6] Early on, training and experience were emphasised. Today, explanatory pictures of the body's inside are common in anatomy, physiology and/or pathology atlases or 'maps' containing pictures of the body's organs, and cells, and are used in health care professionals' curricula. Similarly to McGrath (2002), Birke (1999) uses the term 'reading' in regard to pictures of the biological body: they 'have to be read' (p. 74), and one must 'learn to read the inside' (p. 71). One must learn how to abstract, to move from the particular to the universal, to compare, and to 'render the image into universal form' (Birke 1999: 59). Novice students learning microscopy *do* see something in the microscope, but:

it is rather that they do not know *how* to see, how to interpret and frame whatever lines and colours fill the field of the view, how to distinguish the 'real' from the artefact, the cell from the air bubble.

(Birke 1999: 59)

Pictures of the body's inside, including cells, are thus not self-explanatory. A core feature of cytology, including the Pap smear, is that the visual analysis of magnified cells is guided by predetermined classifications and involves the distinction between, and identification of, cells in a continuum between the normal and the pathological.

The normal, the pathological and the spectrum between

The concept of 'the normal' is used across disciplinary borders. Normality can be defined in different ways for different purposes, e.g. statistical or clinical (Posner 1993). In medicine, 'the normal' has been defined as agreeing with the regular and established type (Dorland and Anderson 1993). About four decades ago Ryle (1961) argued that the meaning of the normal, which is often equated with healthy, is problematic in biomedicine. According to Ryle the conceptualisation of the normal is unclear since variations of the normal have received less interest and attention than the measurements of disease. Birke (1999), a feminist biologist, points out that 'physiological systems assume a "typical" or "normal" individual' (p. 27). For Birke the notion of the pathological is the most problematic, claiming that in modern biomedical texts deviations from the normal are consistently represented as 'pathological' rather than as 'differences'. Thus, from different angles Ryle (1961) and Birke (1999) problematise the possibilities for variations within the categories of the normal and the pathological, raising questions about at which point the one is transformed into the other.

The Pap smear

The Pap smear epitomizes what has been described as the core features of 'surveillance medicine': the problematisation of the normal and the blurring of the binary relation between the normal and the pathological (Armstrong 1995). As is the case with most screening tests, Pap smears 'yield continuous variables' with a gradual transition from normal to morbid conditions (Swedish Council on Technology Assessment in Health Care 1996: 13). As mentioned, Pap smears are analysed in a continuum between the normal and the pathological using the microscope and a cytological classification systems. Whereas the term classifications connote fixed categories, Pap smear classifications have been in a state of flux. According to Clarke and Casper (1996), the Papanicolaou classification system has undergone 'several incarnations over time' (p. 607). In addition, a variety of conceptualisations have been used in the literature concerning the cells in between the normal and the pathological that are detected by means of the Pap smear. For example, Armstrong (1995) labelled the abnormal cells detected through screening a 'semi-pathological pre-illness at-risk state' (p. 402). In medicine, CIN (cervical intraepithelial neoplasia) has been described as 'a single diagnostic category' and 'a single disease continuum' into which 'all pre-malignant epithelial abnormalities' are put (Robertson 1989: 273).

Classificatory systems and boundaries have also been of interest to social scientists (e.g. Douglas 1979, Star and Griesemer 1989, Clarke and Casper 1996). In her classical text Douglas (1979) has shown that classifications should be analysed and related to cultural contexts and involve notions about order and disorder. According to Douglas classifications can be seen as a sorting process, and as part of the creation and maintenance of some kind of order. This order centrally includes the labelling of objects. The labelling as such affects how objects are perceived since 'once labelled they are more speedily slotted into the pigeon-holes in future' (ibid.: 36). Although there is a kind of 'conservative bias built in' as 'we make a greater and greater investment in our system of labels' (ibid.: 36), classifications may also be subject to change and modification. For example, the discovery of ambiguous species may create disorder, and disorder spoils patterns. Adopting such an analytic approach, combined with ethnographic methodology, allows one to move beyond ideas about classifications as static taxonomies and to explore the dynamics and meanings that evolve in the daily work with classifications in a clinical medical context.

In the empirical section that follows I will describe how cytological analysis and classification is performed, exemplified by quotes and field notes from both Cyto lab and City lab (pseudonyms for the public and private lab). I will start by showing the meaning of the term *screening*, which captures the cytodiagnosticians' expertise and skills in cytology. I will then describe two main aspects of screening: the *biological mapping of cells* and the *enculturalisation*[7] *of cells*. Finally, the cytodiagnosticians in this study presented themselves as highly aware of the interpretative nature of cytological classifications and also of ways in which such aspects of screening could be handled.

Screening cytology down the microscope as (em)bodied seeing

The cytodiagnosticians at both labs defined screening cytological samples, including the Pap smears, as looking at *all* cells (or the *whole* material) on the *whole* microscope slide, as exemplified below by Anna and Pia, two cytodiagnosticians at Cyto lab:

> Yes, you must look at all of the cells, you must look at all of the material. That's screening.

> Many cytodiagnosticians firmly believe that there are more than fifty or seventy thousand cells on the slide. And you must check everything.

'Looking at everything' was a common term in daily talk about screening. The cytodiagnosticians above also talked about 'checking' everything, or 'looking through' the whole material. However, screening did not mean looking at one cell at a time. Rather, screening meant looking at several cells at once, in a field of vision and for a short amount of time. One such field of vision could contain hundreds of cells, as described by Filippa at Cyto lab:

> In each field of vision you see maybe a hundred, two hundred, three hundred cells or maybe more. But you must be able to see all of them, get an overview and scan the picture with between a hundred to three hundred cells, maybe more. I don't know, I have never counted them – in just a fraction of a second, you know. A tenth or a hundredth of a second, I don't know. Assess and scan all the cells at once. You could never go through every field one by one. That's why it's called 'screening', to screen the cells.

The speed with which the cytodiagnosticians performed screening was said to be highly individual and not possible to increase or reduce on demand. Several informants also said that screening cytology actually *demanded* a certain speed. Hanna, one of the cytodiagnosticians at City lab, described screening as 'a rhythm' she came into:

> You da, da, da, da and then back and forth. It can't be too slow because then you think that everything looks strange. Then you sit and fiddle around and look and find loads of strange cells that aren't really there. You work just as fast even though you don't have much to do.

Thus, even if Hanna had few samples to screen she did not reduce her screening speed, as this did not improve screening. Sarah, a cytodiagnostician at Cyto lab, talked about screening in terms of a 'smooth flow':

> ... when you sit down, then you get a second wind with screening. It flows better after a while.

Every screener had to learn her or his personal screening speed, as it was considered to be highly individual. Also, the speed was not the same for all samples, but varied, as some samples took longer to screen. Although screening speed was commonly acknowledged as something that could not be increased by force or on demand, and was seldom talked about in normative terms, screening speed was not unimportant in either of the labs. For example, both labs had standards for how quickly they would deliver sample notification to the health care facilities (called 'reporting time'). At Cyto lab, fast screeners were appreciated in the sense that they were able to 'really get through work'. The cytodiagnosticians felt some (varied) degree of pressure to keep reporting time during periods of heavy workload. They could not, however, increase their screening speed on demand as this was an individual ability, and as meticulousness was emphasised as *the* most important aspect of screening. It should be noted, however, that a large influx of cytology samples was not merely seen as negative. One of the major components in becoming skilled in cytology, according to all cytodiagnosticians, was to 'see much' and screen a large number of cytology samples.

The cytodiagnosticians performed screening while sitting down. Their head and neck were kept still, and the upper body was tilted slightly forward, with their underarms resting directly on the desk, on arm supports with 'sheepskin', or on sheepskin directly on the table. This position was something all my informants had become accustomed to, although they remembered many kinds of difficulties in the beginning, as described by Anna at Cyto lab:

> ... before one got used to microscopy, on the whole. Sitting and keeping your head still and (...) Setting the ocular correctly and (...) Above all holding your head still. I usually lean a little, against this, so that I have a hollow here under my right eye. I get a little support ...

Screening cytology meant looking straight forward, fixing the eyes in the middle while seeing the cells with their wide-angle vision, and keeping one's head and eyes still, while moving and stopping the slide with a steering control on the microscope stage. During screening, it was necessary to have a sharply focused picture of the cells. The sharpness was adjusted continuously during screening with the focusing control on the microscope (which was moved back and forth with fine-tuned dexterity): for example, when the cells were laying on top of each other instead of as a single layer (called 'monolayer' in the lab vernacular). The sharpness in the microscope was adjusted in order to scrutinise the cells at the different levels of depth on the microscope slide. This adjustment during screening was often described as an 'inbuilt routine'.

Besides looking at all cells by means of adjusting the sharpness of the picture, the cytodiagnosticians did what they called 'overlapping'. Overlapping was described as a compulsory 'system' or a 'routine' to look at all the cells, which was accomplished by moving the slide back and forth between the edges of the slide, and very slightly sideward, in a zig-zag movement while always keeping one part of the previous field of vision within the new one:

> ... in fact, you look at all of the cells twice. Because you must work all the time with a little 'overlapping', it's called overlapping. You go first straight over the slide, turn, and move [the microscope slide] a little to the side. And then straight over the slide again, and then move it when you get to the edge up and down the slide. You have to have a system, so that you can look at *all* of the cells (...) now I have gone right across

so I have to move the slide a little, in one direction. So that I see *all* the cells and from the beginning to the end, there'll be about thirty-seven, thirty-six, thirty-eight turns. If you don't overlap then you can miss the edge there every time.

(Diana, City lab)

Overlapping was a technique used to ensure that the cytodiagnosticians saw all the cells on the slide during screening. If not properly conducted they could miss cells in the intermediary zone. This aspect of screening, described below by Isabel, a cytodiagnostician at Cyto lab, was in fact stressed by all the cytodiagnosticians:

... it [the overlapping] is very important, there can be one cell on the whole slide, and it can lie in between too, so it's very important ...

Overlapping was said to 'go by itself' and similarly to adjusting sharpness its procedure was not consciously considered during screening, as exemplified by Beatrice at Cyto lab and Sophie at City lab:

... I just go, I have overlapping programmed into my body, in my fingertips.

... I must make the overlap ten, fifteen per cent (...) When you are so experienced as we are, then you know exactly how much you are going to jump. I sort of *feel* it, it's in my fingers.

Sophie, the second cytodiagnostician above, explained that overlapping was defined as an exact percentage. However, she did not make a mathematical calculation every time she did the zig-zag movement with the steering control. As shown above, by experience overlapping became understood as felt and situated in the cytodiagnosticians' fingers. One of my informants, Yvonne, who had been a cytodiagnostician for over thirty years, explained that she had once tried a device (that was put on the microscope) to mechanically regulate overlapping. She was generally fond of and welcomed all kinds of new technology in her work. However, this device was not of any help as it made the microscope stiff. She realised that she did not need the device:

YVONNE: ... It was so sluggish because then the whole microscope becomes like a threshing machine (...) and then you notice, you do it anyway, because you see it when you move. So then you see when the one cell is at the other end so to speak. So you do it automatically.
ANETTE: So you don't jump sort of a few centimetres?
YVONNE: No, no, oh no. You don't do that you see. And then we counted when we had that machine. Because that did, I think it was thirty-eight

times that it said 'click, click, click'. And then you screen yourself and then you count how many times you did it approximately, and it was the same thing. You have it in your eyes.

Several experienced cytodiagnosticians emphasised the value of ergonomic improvements of the microscope. Present microscopes are much better adapted to the body, as compared with those in the 1960s, they said. Basically, the microscope was the tool that enabled them to 'enter another world' and seemed for many of them to have become an extension of their bodies:

> This [the microscope] is my 'tool of the trade', it should be clean and it should be properly set up, and it should not be defective in any way. It is my eyes ...
>
> (Petra, Cyto lab)

> It is a world of colours and cells (...) the microscope is sort of a device that takes me into this world. Without the microscope I can't get into this world.
>
> (Filippa, Cyto lab)

> ... It means a lot to have a good microscope, which has good magnification and that you feel comfortable with and sit well with (...) It becomes almost personal. You have to have your own in order to feel good and not get problems. It is immediately noticeable if someone else has sat there ...
>
> (Birgitta, Cyto lab)

The diagnosticians had learned screening by a bodily socialisation. First, they often emphasised how screening 'should be done', in talk and practice, according to shared and commonly accepted criteria (e.g. to look at everything, the importance of overlapping and the adjusting of sharpness). Second, the cytodiagnosticians skills in screening cytology can be conceptualised as (em)bodied seeing where the microscope had become an extension of their bodies. They no longer consciously thought about how to handle the microscope, how to look at all cells on the microscope slide, when and how to make the picture sharp, with what speed they should perform screening, and finally how to do overlapping. However, not all aspects of screening were embodied in the above-mentioned sense. Assessing the representativeness of the samples or performing screening with a new microscope where examples of more consciously performed screening, even after long experience. I indicate both aspects by putting 'em' in embodied in brackets.

The (biological) mapping of cells

During screening the cytodiagnosticians made a visual sorting of the cytology samples by assessing and distinguishing between normal and (potentially) non-normal cells. Whereas their diagnostic responsibility was 'normal' cervical cytology, or as they also say 'benign' cytology (I will use the terms interchangeably), they also marked potentially non-normal cells with the 'dotting thing' (laboratory vernacular for the marking objective on the microscope) and suggested a diagnosis. The cytodiagnosticians had a refined and differentiated vocabulary for both normal cells and cells that deviated from the normal and often pointed at a list containing what they referred to as predetermined 'diagnoses', 'groups', 'classes' or 'codes' representing scientific cytological knowledge about cells. These lists were often kept at hand during screening, as shown by Anita at Cyto lab:

> ... see for yourself how many different diagnoses we have. There really are a lot [she turns towards her desk and shows a paper] and then to match it right, yes maybe it was only one side (...) No, here you have almost two pages.

When elaborating on these predetermined classifications my informants said they represented various *types* of cells, for example 'squamous' or 'glandular' cells. The classifications also represented normality, or *degrees* of deviations referred to as 'CIN I', 'CIN II' and 'CIN III' that 'originally belonged' to different cell layers:

> ... you can find dysplasias, atypias, as you also call them, that is different types of, degrees of atypia that you can see in cells depending on which layer of cells and how much they are changed (...) There's an old grading of mild atypia, moderate atypia, severe atypia, CIN I, CIN II, and CIN III (...) and as I learned CIN I, it is usually the surface cells, superficial cells, mostly, and then moderate atypia, CIN II, it is mostly those intermediate cells, if they are atypical. It is not so easy. You learn after a while that they are intermediate cells and if it's ugly then it must be moderate atypia, or CIN II (...) and then CIN III are those there, most lowest part or parabasal cells, you usually see that they show atypia. If you discover that it *is*, must be, parabasal cells so it *is* CIN III. The quantity doesn't make much difference in this context. It is the type of cells ...
>
> (Filippa, Cyto lab)

The diagnosticians not only classified cervical cells in regard to normality and deviance. They assessed and classified cells in regard to hormone cyclical changes and patterns on the slide. They could not *see* the hormones, only their effects on the cells. They also assessed and classified various species that were present on the slide, or had affected the cells on the slide. Even though cytology is not a method to classify bacteria, as my informants said, they could see and interpret typical affects on cells caused by several micro-organisms. Thus, the cells were interpreted in relation to their 'natural environment' as presented on each slide:

> As soon as I put the slide in here, I can react immediately 'Aha!' Now this patient doesn't have it but 'Oh dear! There are cocci here' ... then my brain thinks 'these cells can be little affected by the cocci' and I must take that into account, when I assess the smear. She has ordinary Döderlein, and that is what is most common, normal (...) doesn't affect the cells. You couldn't say that.
>
> (Cecilia, Cyto lab)

Classifications of cells were thus quintessential in my informants' work with screening cytology. A crucial aspect of classifications was also that they provided a basis for medical treatment of the patient, as described by Marit at City lab:

> Yes, of course you must have classifications because you treat the patient in different ways depending on what they have, what diagnosis they get.

When the cytodiagnosticians learned screening they first became accustomed to and learnt to identify normal cytology. Normality did not speak for itself. It is notable that even normality was part of an active classificatory process.

> You get to make a diagnosis, even if it is only benign, you get to take a stand. It makes it more fun ...
>
> (Hanna, City lab)

Most of them said that long experience had given them a picture of the normal 'in their head', as described below by Ingegerd at City lab (first quote) and Anita at Cyto lab (second quote):

> We've learned what a benign cell should look like. Yes, it's in your head.

> ... I have the normal somewhere in my head. I have seen it. I know how it should look when it's normal and then I compare all the time, the new cells that I see with the normal. That's the way it has to be, or? [laugh] I haven't really thought about it so much, how to express it, and yes, put it into words. I just *see* that it is like that, and then of course you could describe it better ...

The cytodiagnosticians above claimed that finding deviant cells and differentiating between normal and atypical cells was something they *saw,* but how they knew by seeing was difficult to verbalise. The manner in which the cytodiagnosticians identified and distinguished between normal and non-normal cells in daily practice was said to be difficult to put into words. Thus, my informants' visual repertoire of cytology was more extended than their verbal repertoire.

Assessments and classification of normal cytology were not made from one single standard of normality for all samples. Instead, the cytodiagnosticians assessed normality in regard to several standards. The standards for classifying cells as normal varied and were dependent on type of series:

> ... you must, in some way, re-arrange your thinking then, that the bladder is different from ascites for example. If you take a bladder sample and look at it and believe that this is ehh a gynaecological sample. Then you just put malignant on it (...) What you are *looking* at and what is it that you are going to look for (...) and how the normal in just this type of sample looks.
>
> (Rose, Cyto lab)

Besides conceiving of normalities in the plural, the diagnostician below also defined non-normal cells as a kind of normality, that is, when for example CIN I cells unequivocally belonged to, or could be fitted into that particular classification – typical CIN I cells, where thus those cells could positively be identified and assigned as 'normal CIN I cells', as described by Hedvig at Cyto lab:

> So there are certain criteria (...) and then certain types of cell that have a particular look. You recognise that there are certain cells you will find here, you look at a cancer for example, and those cells are normal when you look at a mild dysplasia. Normal, so to speak, ordinary you can say maybe. They are not normal. In mild dysplasia, it is so that there are no normal cells, there are atypical cells but they are normal for this picture. That is, so that you assess, 'aha this is a typical CIN I', or, 'these are mildly dysplastic cells'.

To positively fit the cells on the slide into one of the predetermined classifications was a crucial part of the assessment process. When the cytodiagnosticians assessed cytology as 'typical', classification went smoothly as the cells with little doubt positively fitted into a particular classification. To assess whether cells positively fitted into one of the classifications was a core feature in daily screening. A salient feature of the uses of classifications was that the cytodiagnosticians were able to 'sift away' all cells, bacteria, artefacts, and so on, as soon as these had been classified. Identifying particular bacteria or cervical glandular cells made it possible to 'disregard' them. By claiming that classifications enable the cytodiagnosticians both to identify and disregard cells (and other features on the slide), I do not mean that they then forgot about what they had found on the slide. On the contrary, they often said that they made a comprehensive assessment of the whole slide when they finished screening the slide. However, the continuous classification of all that was present on the slide during screening allowed the cytodiagnosticians to proceed. They could for example rather quickly classify a group of cells as CIN I cells, mark them with the 'dotting thing' ('prickmoj' in Swedish), and continue screening the slide. The process whereby cells, bacteria and even artefacts positively fitted into a classification thus made it possible to 'disregard' them for the moment, and proceed with screening, looking for other cells that were similar to, or different from those already classified. When this process went smoothly, it took only about five minutes to screen the cervical cytology slide. However, if they were unable to classify what they saw, they would also use the dotting thing, but would get stuck on this group of cells: perhaps they would have to ask a colleague for advice. The process of reaching an unequivocal accord between cells (and other features) and classifications is clearly described in the example below during screening:

> Well, I look at the age, and then I know approximately how it should look. I see the bacteria at once. When you put the slide under the microscope, then you see what kind of bacteria there is, and then you can put it aside. Yes, well (...) when I've decided what kind of bacteria it is, then I can sort it out of the way. If I've seen that there are glandular cells, that should be there, then I put it aside. Then it's only the ugly cells (...) Yes, now I looked at this request form and it says there that she is born –26 and takes no hormones. And then the sample should look in a particular way. You have dry mucous membranes. You see that right away, because it kind of fits. If she had looked like a young girl, yes another kind of picture, then you would have reacted and thought it was wrong, or if she takes hormones. But, it almost always fits when you put in the slide, and then you don't think any more of it. She has no bacteria, so I don't have to think more about *that*. This one is born –58 and she has an IUD [intrauterine contraceptive device], and then they usually have a lot of inflammatory cells, a foreign thing in the body. And she has! It's inflamed. It's probably not something she notices (...) and then I go down and look at what's there, and there were cocci, they often have them, those with IUDs. So, there are a lot of leucocytes.

An interesting issue about the relation between classifications, knowledge and seeing was raised when the cytodiagnosticians discussed changes in the general picture of cells over the years. For example, there was a consensus that HPV (human papilloma virus) had increased and trichomonas and herpes had almost disappeared. It was thought that eventually new cytodiagnosticians would rarely see trichomonas. A tricky question raised by my informants was whether today's common existence of HPV was a 'real' increase, or if it had been present earlier. Some said it was possible that HPV had been there for a long time, but that the role of HPV, some types of which are strongly associated with cervical cancer, and its effects in on cells had not become part of their knowledge and their visual repertoire until recently.

The cytodiagnosticians' work with the Pap smear thus involves, and indeed presupposes, knowledge about the 'biological order' of cells. A central feature of screening and assessing the Pap smear involves positively matching that which was seen on the slide to predetermined classifications. That which can be classified with little interpretative efforts can also be 'un-seen', rendered part of the background and thus enable the cytodiagnostician to proceed with screening. Whereas the relationship between cells and classifications seems to be circular: the cytodiagnosticians classify the cells that they see on the slide, and they see that which they are able to classify, neither the classifications used for classifying cells nor the cells present on the slide have been stable over time. However, there is more to say about cells and classifications in a cytology laboratory context.

Enculturalising cells

Thus far, I have described the (biological) mapping of cells, that is, the interpretative process whereby the predetermined classifications – the biological map of cells – were applied onto cells on the microscope slides. I will continue to describe notions that exist in addition to the biological mapping of cells related to: (i) cells that are difficult or impossible to classify – cells that are at the margins of classifications; and (ii) the perfect match, which is rare, between cells and classifications.

Cells at the margins of classifications

In daily practice the cells of cytology samples may also be unclear, difficult and at times even impossible to classify, which is the focus of this section.

> During the demm [the labs vernacular for the joint diagnostic session in the multi-headed microscope] a cytologist, a cytodiagnostician, and a physician in training are assessing cervical cytology. The cytologist scrutinizes the dots on the slide marked by the cytodiagnostician. He then says 'this is a slight CIN I'. He explains that he has to choose something that is clear and concise for the clinicians, or else they would be confused. The next sample is suggested by the cytodiagnostician to be a CIN III. The cytologist considers it however to be a CIN II. He also says that when a cytologist's and a cytodiagnostician's assessment differ by two steps, another cytologist would be asked to assess the sample.

During another demm, another cytologist and cytodiagnostician are assessing indicated cervical cytology. The cytologist takes a cytology request form and the two adjacent slides. The cytodiagnostician says that apparently gynaecologists nowadays sometimes take two slides for the indicated cervical cytology samples. The cytologist assesses the dots in silence, and then says: 'this is zero point five', and laughs. He then takes the second slide of the two, which he also assesses in silence. After a while he says: 'this one is one point twenty-five'.

In the two cases above from different joint diagnostic sessions at Cyto lab (called the 'demm' in the lab vernacular), the cytologists seemed to actually perceive nuances, i.e. further classifications, within the predetermined classifications. This was also the case for the cytodiagnosticians. Whereas the cytologists and the cytodiagnosticians generally considered the predetermined classifications to be adequate for use in daily practice, they said that at times the cells did not match, or fell in between, the classifications, as exemplified by Filippa at Cyto lab:

> You can go across the boundaries too, if you think that (...) you call it CIN I II for example, or CIN II–III. You can call it that, or that's what they do also, and then you mean that most of it, is maybe a CIN I, but there are also cells, cell changes, that are CIN II. It is something like 'What should I do?' If you really don't want to finalise this as a CIN II, but you see that there are cells that *can* be CIN II, then you do this, CIN I–II. That works. So, no, I think that on the whole it is good with the classes that exist.

Others said that occasionally cells were completely impossible to classify. Not all cells could be matched with a particular classification, as the variation of cells exceeded the classifications:

> ... sometimes it just doesn't work, to put it simply, there aren't codes so that it agrees.
>
> (Karin, Cyto lab)

Another cytodiagnostician raised this point as well:

ELSA: Sometimes it just doesn't work to say 'what is this here?', I just see that the cells are changed, that there is something that isn't normal.
ANETTE: It doesn't always work to fit it into the classification system?
ELSA: No, no, no. You see that the cells are changed by bacteria, or candida or trichomonas, or (...) but you *know* that picture, so to speak. But then there is yes, that sometimes the cells are badly preserved, or unclear in some other way, and then they often come in those groups. Ehh (...) unclear, new sample, for the sake of safety, so to speak.

The classificatory system was generally believed to cover almost all cases. No one wanted another system or wanted to add new classifications when I asked them about it. Thus, the system used at the labs in terms of pre-determined diagnoses was seen as a valuable tool, but was not claimed to perfectly or unambiguously mirror and represent the entire variation of cells on the slides. The predetermined classifications and the picture of cells under the microscope were not always possible to match.

Sometimes there were pragmatic reasons for the inability to classify cells, e.g. that the cells were of bad quality or destroyed. However, when the assessment did not match any of the classifications, or when the diagnosticians were unable to determine type of cell and/or degree of deviance, they could write a classificatory suggestion accompanied with a question mark. As exemplified below by Andrea at Cyto lab, they could also suggest a specific classification for cells that were unclear, difficult, or impossible to classify:

> But you see, there is a lot that is unclear: 'unclear squamous atypia', 'squamous atypia of indeterminate significance'. There are a lot that doesn't work to put in, if there were only those three groups [CIN I, II, III] it would be *really* good. But there is always (...) here you have 'glandular atypia', '*suspicious* of adenocarcinoma', and 'adenocarcinoma', 'unclear atypia', 'unclear' (...) but you can always put it into one of those groups, I think ...

Diagnosticians at both labs had particular names for these classifications:

> It is part of the training that we, you must decide. There are diagnoses which are sort of a 'no-mans-land', 'unclear changes', yes some of those 'slops cases'. Some maybe feel more for them than others do.
>
> (Alice, Cyto lab)

> Sometimes it can be very difficult to determine a diagnosis. It's incredibly difficult, it's difficult for everyone. Then you have that little slops group, difficult to assess (laughs) ... Or, atypia of uncertain significance. You don't really know ...
>
> (Diana, City lab)

> ... there are many such unclear cases. It can be glandular cells that are lying on top of each other so that they look a little darker. Then you have all those that are (...) aren't simple. They end up in unclear, in the slops pail and in that [group] there are the completely benign and there are the really bad. Then it is so (...) that the doctor treating them doesn't ignore (...) There are a lot of very difficult cases. There is an awful lot of rubbish there that are completely benign but there are also a lot that are cancer ...
>
> (Hillevi, Cyto lab)

So, there seemed to be something else going on simultaneously with the scientific knowledge and the biological mapping of cells in relation to unclassifiable cells. The prefix used by my informants: 'slops', can be interpreted as relating to the clash between the *imperative* and the *impossibility* to classify all cells. This diagnostic category was sometimes necessary in daily cytology laboratory practice, which is characterised by a struggle to separate and classify cells according to normality, cancer and the degrees in between. However, although unclassifiable cells were kept in some control by being classified *qua* unclassifiable, this group could contain a potentially 'dangerous' mix of both normal and pathological cells. As such, the group containing unclassifiable cells disrupts order and threatens the mandate of the cytology laboratory. However, the daily work with assessing cells also involved cases where the match between the cells and the classifications were perfectly clear.

Exceptional matching of cells and classifications

It is half an hour past demm's scheduled start at Cyto lab. The cytodiagnostician who has demm looks for the cytologist responsible for the demm today who is late. He arrives and takes a seat at his usual place by the main ocular in the middle. The cytodiagnostician takes a seat in the usual place in front of the cytologist slightly to the left by the computer screen ready to use the mouse. Today two other physicians under training also participate. One of them sits beside the cytodiagnostician and the other one sits to the right of the cytologist. First, there are a number of samples that the cytologist assesses as normal. He informs the physicians under training about the predetermined 'standard codes' and says they cover 90 per cent of the cases. During the demm he mostly uses these standard codes, but in some cases he formulates a diagnosis verbally in the dictating machine, using his own words. The cytologist has a formal and slightly jocular manner and encourages the new physicians to express their opinion and to argue with him. He asks the physicians several times 'What is your opinion?' or 'Do you agree?' When the physicians under training make their suggestions he says 'I trust you …'. Now and then they ask the cytologist to explain further by saying 'Can you please …' or 'Excuse me …'. While assessing the samples he tells the physicians under training about other possible interpretations and about various forms of cancers. He tells them about some types of cytology that are particularly difficult to assess. Suddenly the three participants protest loudly, and the cytologist says: 'Excuse me'. He had just taken the same cytology request form twice by mistake. The cytodiagnostician is asked several times to display the patients' previous test results on the screen, and to read them out loud. On one occasion, when the cytologist is about to assess a sample he considers normal, the cytodiagnostician says loudly to the cytologist: 'You cannot let this one go!' After some discussion he agrees and decides to follow her advice. Suddenly, the cytologist calls out: 'This is beautiful! This one we must add to the collection'. The others agree. The 'beautiful' sample is said to be colon cancer.

During another daily demm with another personnel group at Cyto lab, the cytologist calls out 'This is beautiful! You should take a picture of this!' They talk about the sample as a 'crystal clear HPV'. The cytodiagnostician turns towards me and says: 'You can see that, can't you?'

The examples from the field notes above derive from two different demm sessions at Cyto lab, out of many, in which there were examples of 'beautiful' cells. The 'beautiful' cells in the two cases seemed to have little in common: the first case was about a type of cancer, and the second case was about signs of HPV (virus). Yet, the participants referred to both cases as 'beautiful'.

In the second case above, the cytodiagnosticians thought that I, a researcher not trained in cytology, might also see what was beautiful in a 'crystal clear' HPV. However, I could not see anything I perceived as 'beautiful', neither with the colon cancer cells nor with the HPV affected cells. All demm sessions I attended occasionally contained samples described as beautiful regardless of whether the assessment concerned normal or malignant cells, or bacteria, candida, or viral effects on cells. For example, during one diagnostic session there was a group of cells that was described as 'very beautiful benign urothelial cells'. To me the same group of cells appeared as round, delineated, dark blue dots that were lying some distance from each other in a regular pattern. As exemplified below by Pia at Cyto lab, beautiful cases were not only talked about during demm:

When you sit two [cytodiagnosticians] in a room, 'Can you look at this?' 'No, look, it is really nice-looking, this CIS.'

The first cytologist in the examples from the demm above talked about adding 'the beautiful colon cancer' to the collection, and the second one talked about taking a picture of the 'crystal clear HPV'. Thus, these beautiful cases were talked about in terms of being *preserved* for some additional purpose. This was a common theme during the demm whenever a 'beautiful' case was determined. But why did some cases merit preservation? What was the difference between these cases and other ones? The cytodiagnosticians occasionally talked about samples that should be preserved, as well:

Yes, we are talking about textbook examples then, that are good to have in a collection.

As described below, expressions like 'collections' and 'textbook examples' seemed to refer to exceptionally clear and typical cases:

When the changes are in the surface cells, in the superficial cells, in the sample. If it's those cells that are not normal, then it is CIN I. And then, if it is deeper, and there are intermediate cells in it, and also superficial cells, then it is CIN II. This is very simplified this here, what I am saying (…) and then if it is *even deeper* down, so that there are *basal cells* in the sample too. First it is superficial cells and intermediates, and basal cells. Then there are parabasal cells (…) and if those cells that sit in the basement layer are changed, then it is CIN III. And then there's also cancer in situ that is more like the whole chunk then. And there are also changes in glandular cells. Then there is cancer, it is difficult to say then, *if* there are glandular cells or squamous cells. Yes, of course you learned that once. How it should be. There are always textbook examples. Like that, like that, like that so, of course there are simple rules to follow.

(Olivia, Cyto lab)

The diagnosticians talked about typical and exceptionally clear cases, for example in regard to cells, bacteria, or indications of virus effect on the cells. Such cases were often referred to as 'clear-cut' or 'classic', for example 'a classic CIN I' or 'clear-cut CIS'. For example, Filippa at Cyto lab described how some viruses, like HPV, could display a very distinct and typical picture of cells:

… you see it, you call it 'birds' eyes' in English. You see clearing around the nucleus in the cytoplasm, which almost looks like a bird's eye, you could say and that is the first sign, that there is clearing around the nucleus. It is often orange cytoplasm. It is a little clear around the nucleus. It has a special appearance.

This may have been the kind of picture that the cytologist saw during the demm in the second of the introductory examples, when he wanted to take a picture of the 'crystal clear HPV'. But how did aesthetic notions such as 'beautiful' relate to this? The easy accessibility and interpretability of the relatively scarce classical samples seemed to have an aesthetic value in themselves – they were deemed 'beautiful' samples. The cytodiagnostician above also talked about the importance of 'seeing it'. A core feature of cytological assessments is that it is quintessential to have visual evidence for one's assessment. The pivotal role of visual evidence was also clear when visual evidence was lacking. At times, the effect on the cells by bacteria, virus or candida was more diffuse. Sometimes a particular classification could be suspected without finding any visible evidence:

Maybe sometimes you don't see it, but you see that it must basically be condyloma. If you see it you are a hundred percent certain that it is that. But sometimes you can maybe get a feeling. It *can* be koilocytes, those changes are called koilocytes …

(Filippa, Cyto lab)

The importance of visual evidence is also clearly displayed in another example that concerns candida:

> And then it could also be, I do that, I don't know, I think there are some others too. You can see 'this patient has candida', and then you don't *find* the candida! And you screen, and screen, and screen but you are one hundred and ten percent convinced that the patient has candida and in the end maybe furthest up somewhere, you find a little bit and it can be a good idea to mark it so that you can go back. Because if that is going to go to after-checking and the person who is going to check me says 'there is no candida', 'oh, yes, of course there is'. They have a very special appearance. They become very fiery in appearance. They have stronger colour (...) a more red colour.

In daily practice cells could display visual evidence of a clear diagnosis, or display only a subtle indication, without visual evidence. A perfect match between the cells and the classifications implied the possibility for unambiguous assessment, and easy cases implied those cases where the match between cells and classification were particularly clear and typical. Thus, I suggest that the similarity between the introductory cases of the beautiful colon cancer and the HPV-affected cells is that the beautiful cells referred to were examples of a perfect and unambiguous match between a particular classification of cells and the picture of cells. 'Beautiful' cells thus encompassed cases where – regardless of diagnosis – the match between the picture of cells and the classification was unambiguous, and importantly, where there was strong visual evidence for the assessment.

The self-classifying classifier

The criteria that the cytodiagosticians had learned during their education – which involved that of 'textbook examples' – were applied on all cells, all slides, every day, and year after year. However, as shown, in daily practice the cells assessed were not always 'textbook examples'. Moreover, the existing criteria, guidelines and pre-determined diagnoses that guided the assessment at the labs, were said to be applicable to 90 per cent of the cases, but they did not randomly land on the cells. The point is also that often when the cytodiagnosticians described how they differentiated between the CIN I, II and III cells, they could talk about classifications or pictures of cells that were more difficult than others, and also about why and what made assessments difficult. They talked about how, when, and what kind of internal and external factors they thought influenced their assessments. A general difficulty in cytological assessment was described by one of the cytodiagnosticians:

ANETTE: But do you have criteria for how you will sort, when you think that it is a CIN II, or CIN III or CIN I?

ALICE: Yes, you have that in-built, but it's fluid you know and specifically when it concerns mild cell changes. On certain days you can be, can be high on the scale [in your diagnosis]. You can refer those that you may be a little doubtful about but then the next day you think: '*That* is really nothing', you don't need to refer that one. You understand, you have different days, and then it depends on how, if you have sat through a demonstration with some doctor who diagnoses a little higher than you are used to. If you have sat through a demonstration with X [name of physician] who diagnoses very low, or, yes, it depends a lot sort of. You calibrate yourself all the time with (...) depending on who you have been at a demonstration with too.

Thus, the borders between cellular classifications were not seen as completely stable, and the border between minor cellular changes and benign cytology was generally described as a particularly 'floating border'. First, note that the cytodiagnostician above talks about her colleagues in terms of 'aiming high' (that is, a tendency of going for higher grades), or 'aiming low' (that is, a tendency of going for lower grades). Second, she 'calibrates' her own assessments against those of her colleagues. 'Calibration' was a strategy that my informants used to 'stabilise' themselves in regard to the relatively fluid border between classificatory categories on the level of cells, and to keep these borders in congruence with common criteria and standards. Examples of calibrating strategies were getting a full night sleep, asking colleagues who could 'counter-balance' their assessment, or, at Cyto lab, by participating in the demm. Some said that when they wanted to discuss their assessments they went to a colleague who was *not* at the same level as themselves. Thus, what at first sight deceptively appeared to be highly isolated work at the microscopes was in fact often highly interactive: as described by Anna at Cyto lab:

> ... so you have your own friends who you go to. The ones you know of. You don't go to someone that you yourself think, it sounds a little harsh this, but you don't go to someone, that you think is worse than yourself. You go to someone who has more experience. You learn quite quickly, how, on a scale of one to five, how, where the person in question, and where you yourself lie. So I know that it doesn't help me to go to some people, I am just as uncertain anyway.

Furthermore, the diagnosticians seemed to keep track of, and compensate for, influences that might have a negative impact on their assessments. Some said that the shape they were in that day influenced what they perceived to be difficult or not, which they claimed was not unique for their group of professionals. Still others talked about their individual 'best time of day' which varied from the morning to the afternoon. One common strategy when samples were difficult to classify was to put the sample aside until the next morning:

> Mmm, this here is an SOI case. Yes, sleep on it. I'll look at that one when I am not tired, it is often best ...
>
> (Maria, Cyto lab)

What was difficult to assess could vary from day to day as well. Regardless of day-to-day variations of cells the cytodiagnosticians were generally clear about what affected these variations and also the general aim of their work:

> ... you have sort of different days too. Sometimes you're maybe a little more alert than other days, you are maybe a little tired some days, can be that it is morning or afternoon. Sometimes late in the afternoon, you find something, vaginal smear, you mark it 'this is something, but I can't decide what'. Ehh, then I leave it until the next day. Everyone does it, more or less. You leave it until the next morning, then you look again. Then it is much clearer, than if you are tired in the afternoon (...) because I certainly want to decide for certain, and I don't think that I am just speaking for myself, but for most of us, nearly all. To be able to decide the right diagnosis from the start, that I sign out the request form on the computer (...) Yes, I want to feel sort of that, when it comes from me, that it will be as correct as possible.
>
> (Beatrice, Cyto lab)

The work with assessing and classifying cells is thus performed by subjects who present themselves as well aware of themselves *qua* classifiers, and as having various strategies for making their interpretations as correct as possible.

Discussion and concluding comments

It is commonly accepted that cytology samples – of which the Pap smear test is perhaps the most widely known – have significance for the detection, diagnosis and/or prevention of cancer diseases. It is perhaps less well known *how* such work is performed. The cytology laboratory is a place where the boundaries of normality, and between normality and abnormality, are established on the level of cells; here cells via the microscope as mediator are interpreted and ascribed cultural meaning, and here the inside of the laboratory and the outside world meet and diverge. Ethnographic approaches are well suited to exploring this work at the site where it is performed.

Assessing and classifying cells, as my fieldwork shows, is more complex than one might assume, and has several layers of meaning. Screening cytology down the microscope, for example, 'embraces the whole body' and involves 'subjective engagement' for better or worse (Okely 2001: 101). For worse, as with any human interpretation in the realm of medicine, it is possible to make mistakes. For better, the cytodiagnosticians present themselves as well aware of the interpretative nature of, and the risks inherent in, classifying cells. It is also notable that in contrast to the previously mentioned distinction made by Cartwright (1995) about 'static' and 'moving' technologies (regarding the co-evolution of medical knowledge and technology), the cytodiagnosticians used the microscope as *both* a static and moving instrument of visualisation.

The challenges in cytological classifications were not the same for all cytodiagnosticians in this study. For some, the main challenge was to be able to correctly fit the cells into classifications, to 'get it exactly right'. For others the main challenge was to keep normal and deviant cells separate, that is, to guard the border between normal and deviant cells. These features of classifications in the cytology laboratory can be related to Douglas (1979). She argues that although classifications are relative to cultural contexts, classifications generally determine what belongs to a particular category, and that which cannot be combined and should be kept apart. Classifications in the cytology laboratory were used in both ways with emphasis either on assigning cells to a predetermined classification or to draw a line between normal and deviant cells. The interpretative process whereby cells that perfectly match are deemed 'beautiful' and those cells that are impossible to classify are deemed 'slops' indicates that something more is going on in the work with cells.

First, although the classifications represent a kind of *biological map* of cells, the map does not randomly land on the cells and does not exactly mirror the entire cellular variation. As in any classificatory system, cytological classification generates its own by-products. The cells that could not be classified were referred to as the 'slops group'. The slops group can be related to Douglas' (1979) discussion on dirt. There is no such thing as absolute dirt, Douglas argues. Dirt is the by-product of order, that which offends order. Even the word 'slops' used for this category of unclear cells connotes garbage or refuse – that is, the dirty in the laboratory world. The significance of dirt involves reflection on the relationship between order and disorder, being and non-being, form and formlessness and even life and death. The cytological classifications thus also produce their own by-products of order, in this ambiguous species that connotes disorder and formlessness. In Douglas' view, ambiguous species created by (all) classificatory processes symbolise both danger and power and have to be controlled. In cytology, cells that are not straightforwardly classifiable – the ambiguous cells – are thus controlled by creating special groups for such cells. However, the 'slops' group may contain a mix of both normal and cancerous cells, and thus constitute danger and a threat to the mandate of the cytology laboratory. Second, in cytology in general, no two slides have an identical amount, composition, and pattern of cells. Therefore it is rare that a picture of cells unambiguously and with little interpretative effort matches a particular predetermined classification or prototypical picture of a particular disease. While assessing cytology during screening and the joint diagnostic sessions (i.e. the 'demm'), the issue implicitly addressed by the enthusiasm surrounding beautiful cases is that cells occasionally provided strong and unambiguous visual evidence for a match between pictures of cells and classifications. Conceptualising something as beautiful by virtue of being exceptional has been described by Brunius (1986) and may be called *the aesthetics of the exceptional*.

To avoid possible misunderstanding, the cytodiagnosticians and the cytologists did not make their assessments based on aesthetic notions. Rather, notions about the beautiful and the slops were communicated in addition to scientific knowledge about cells during assessment and classification. This repertoire can, on the one hand, be seen as esoteric: only a limited group, including cytodiagnosticians and cytologists, can see the beautiful in an exceptionally clear 'CIS' or 'colon cancer'. On the other hand, it can also be argued that the biological notions of the body expand to the realm of the social when technologies are used to classify cells. Also, by means of cytology and the classification systems used in the daily assessment of cells, the realm of the social – which is commonly assumed to be outside and external to the body – 'enters' the cells in the biological body. As such, cytology, including the Pap smear and its classifications provides an excellent entry point to problematise the notion that the biological body – composed of billions of cells, that are only accessible via medical technology, i.e. a host of representational manipulations, and fundamental to Western biomedicine – constitutes a black box, or a tabula rasa that tells us brute facts about the normal and the pathological. Cytological classifications can be said to exemplify Lloyd's (1998) arguments that first, human judgement on health and disease in general inevitably involves questions of classifications, and second, classifications about normality and abnormality are not simply 'extracted' from organisms. The organism *itself* will not tell us what counts as the ideal functions. Paraphrasing Hannerz (1996), between our cells and what we know about them, 'there is an information gap, and we fill that gap with culture' (p. 35). What counts as normal involves human judgement, although it is commonly assumed that science informs us about what is normal or abnormal, diseased or healthy, and that 'the social and moral issues begin where the science leaves off' (Lloyd 1998: 552). In cytological assessments, 'living organisms' and 'living people' (Ingold 1990) do not form mutually exclusive realms, as in order for a cytodiagnostician to answer the question 'What's in a Pap smear?' biology, culture, technology and self constitute intersecting realms.

Acknowledgements

Gareth Morgan and Ulla-Liina Lehtinen have provided valuable support in an early draft of this chapter. Economic support for this work has been gratefully received from the Swedish Foundation for Health Care Sciences and Allergy Research (Vårdalstiftelsen), and from the Board of Research for Health and Caring Sciences, the Board of Postgraduate Education, and the Division of Nursing, all at Karolinska Institutet.

Notes

1 Papanicolaou had initial difficulties in gaining acceptance of his method. Casper and Clarke (1998) claim that the adoption and widespread use of the Pap smears relied on a number of initiatives, alliances and power struggles whereby the Pap smear was made 'the right tool for the job' of cancer screening.

2 In the USA the figure is over 50 million (Bristow and Montz 2000).

3 Cytology refers to the study of cells, their origin, structure, function and pathology (Dorland and Anderson 1993). In a cytology laboratory context, the Pap smear constitutes *one* form of cytology out of several others (e.g. sputum, bladder washings and breast cytology).

4 The personnel involved in the daily work with the cytology samples are: the lab auxiliaries, the cytodiagnosticians (biomedical technologists with an additional six months training), and the lab physicians (physicians with additional training in cytology and/or pathology). The lab auxiliaries perform most of the routine preparatory work with the cytology samples prior to and after screening and diagnosis. In Sweden, the cytodiagnosticans' main areas of responsibility are 'preparation' and 'screening' of all cytology samples. They are responsible for 'reporting out' *normal* cervical cytology. They are also responsible for discovering, marking (with the marking objective) and suggesting diagnosis of potentially abnormal cells. Thus, if there are any potential abnormal cells on the microscope slide, the cytodiagnosticians are the ones who detect them. The number of abnormal cells on a slide varies and can, in some cases, be only a handful. The lab physicians are responsible for the final diagnosis of all abnormal/ pathological cells, which they perform either individually (the private lab, here called 'City lab', used this system), or together with one of the cytodiagnosticians by the multi-headed microscope (the public lab, here called 'Cyto lab', used this system which they called 'demm'). The choice of laboratories was based on some initially known variations: (i) private ownership and county council run laboratories; (ii) the size of the laboratories; and (iii) the number of cervical cytology samples handled. In addition, according to the Swedish National Board of Health and Welfare (1998: 42), there are significant differences between cytology labs in Sweden, concerning, for example, the proportions of deviant samples, the number of dysplasias found, and the proportions of samples that cannot be assessed. According to the National Board of Health and Welfare (ibid.), the large differences in proportions of deviant samples depend on divergences in assessment criteria. The two chosen labs varied in regard to all points. In this chapter, I focus on the cytodiagnosticians and to a lesser degree on the lab physicians. The analysed data represents different persons and both labs. An exception here is the field notes on the joint diagnostic sessions (which was only used at the public lab: 'Cyto lab').

5 See for example *The Report of the Cervical Cancer Inquiry* (1988), and Coney (1988) on the longitudinal study on women with abnormal cervical smears, the aim of which was to prove that carcinoma in situ is not (invariably) a pre-malignant disease, performed at National Women's Hospital, Auckland, New Zealand. A more recent example comes from the United Kingdom (Houston *et al.* 2001) where an external re-screening of 81,000 cervical smears was undertaken in the mid-1990s and where 3,469 women had to undergo a re-check after being

informed that their smears were 'inadequate for accurate reporting' (p. 108). In the New Zealand study the laboratory personnel's diagnoses seem to have been challenged and overruled by one of the clinicians. In the British case the laboratory personnel were involved in screening errors and part of a network described as far from optimal. I have found no documentation of cervical cancer screening failures in Sweden.

6   Bennet, J.H. (1862) *An introduction to clinical medicine*, pp. 106–7. Quoted in McGrath (2002).

7   I have borrowed this term from the sociologist Karin Knorr Cetina (2001).

References

Armstrong, D. (1995) 'The rise of surveillance medicine', *Sociology of Health and Illness*, 17: 393–404.

Babes, A. (1928/1967) 'Diagnosis of cancer of the uterine cervix by smears', Translation from French by L.E. Douglass, *Acta Cytologica*, 1967, 11: 217–23.

Birke, L. (1999) *Feminism and the biological body*, Edinburgh: Edinburgh University Press.

Bristow, R.E. and Montz, F.J. (2000) 'Workup of the abnormal Pap test', *Clinical Cornerstone*, 3: 12–24.

Brunius, T. (1986) *Estetik förr och nu* [Aesthetics in the past and present], Stockholm: Liber.

Butler, S., Nuttall, R.H. and Brown, O. (1986) *The social history of the microscope*, Cambridge: Whipple Museum of the History of Science.

Cartwright, L. (1995) *Screening the body: tracing medicine's visual culture*, Minneapolis, MN: University of Minnesota Press.

Casper, M.J. and Clarke, A.E. (1998) 'Making the Pap smear into the "right tool" for the job: cervical cancer screening in the USA, circa 1940–95', *Social Studies of Science*, 28/2: 255–90.

Clarke, A.E. and Casper, M.J. (1996) 'From simple technology to complex arena: classification of Pap smears, 1917–90', *Medical Anthropology Quarterly*, 10: 601–23.

Coney, S. (1988) *The unfortunate experiment*, Auckland: Penguin.

Dorland, W.A.N. and Anderson, D.M. (1993) *Dorland's illustrated medical dictionary*, Philadelphia, PA: Saunders.

Douglas, M. (1966/1979) *Purity and danger: an analysis of concepts of pollution and taboo*, London: Routledge and Kegan Paul.

Fox Keller, E. (1996) 'The biological gaze', in Robertson, G., Mash, M., Tickner, L., Bird, J., Curtis, B. and Putnam, T. (eds) *Futurenatural: nature, science, culture*, London: Routledge.

Hannerz, U. (1996) 'When culture is everywhere', in *Transnational connections: culture, people, places*, London: Routledge.

Houston, D.M., Lloyd, K., Drysdale, S. and Farmer, M. (2001) 'The benefits of uncertainty: changes in women's perceptions of the cervical screening programme as a consequence of screening errors by Kent and Canterbury NHS trust', *Psychology, Health and Medicine*, 6: 107–13.

Ingold, T. (1990) 'An anthropologist looks at biology', *Man*, 25: 208–29.

Keating, P. and Cambrosio, A. (2000) 'Real compared to what? Diagnosing leukemias and lymphomas', in Lock, M., Young, A. and Cambrosio, A. (eds) *Living and working with the new medical technologies: intersections of inquiry*, Cambridge: Cambridge University Press.

Knorr Cetina, K. (2001) 'Laboratory studies: historical perspectives', in Smelser, N.J. and Baltes, P.B. (eds) *International encyclopedia of the social and behavioral sciences*, Amsterdam: Elsevier, pp. 8232–8.

Knorr Cetina, K. and Amann, K. (1990) 'Image dissection in natural scientific inquiry', *Science, Technology and Human Values*, 15: 259–83.

Koss, L.G. (1989) 'The Papanicolaou test for cervical cancer detection: a triumph and a tragedy', *Journal of the American Medical Association*, 261: 737–43.

Latour, B. and Woolgar, S. (1986) *Laboratory life: the social construction of scientific facts*, Beverly Hills, CA: Sage.

Lloyd, E.A. (1998) 'Normality and variation: the Human Genome Project and the ideal human type', in Hull, D.L. and Ruse, M. (eds) *The philosophy of biology*, Oxford: Oxford University Press.

Lynch, M. (1985) 'Discipline and the material form of images: an analysis of scientific visibility', *Social Studies of Science*, 15: 37–66.

Lynch, M. (1988) 'Sacrifice and the transformation of the animal body into a scientific object: laboratory culture and ritual practice in the neurosciences', *Social Studies of Science*, 18: 265–89.

McGrath, R. (2002) *Seeing her sex: medical archives and the female body*, Manchester: Manchester University Press.

Mol, A. (2000) 'Pathology and the clinic: an ethnographic presentation of two atheroscleroses', in Lock, M., Young, A. and Cambrosio, A. (eds) *Living and working with the new medical technologies: intersections of inquiry*, Cambridge: Cambridge University Press.

Morris, K.A., Kavanagh, A.M. and Gunn J.M. (2001) 'Management of women with minor abnormalities of the cervix detected through screening: a qualitative study', *Medical Journal of Australia*, 174: 126–9.

Nader, L. (1972) 'Up the anthropologist: perspective gained from Studying Up', in Hymes, D. (ed.) *Reinventing anthropology*, New York: Pantheon Books.

Okely, J. (2001) 'Visualism and the landscape: looking and seeing in Normandy', *Ethnos*, 66: 99–120.

Papanicolaou, G.N. (1928) *New cancer diagnosis*, Third Race Betterment Conference. Battle Creek, MI: Race Betterment Foundation.

Posner, T. (1993) 'Ethical issues and the individual woman in cancer screening programmes', *Journal of Advances in Health and Nursing Care*, 2: 55–69.

Rabinow, P. (1996) *Making PCR: a story of biotechnology*, Chicago, IL: University of Chicago Press.

Rapp, R. (1999) *Testing women, testing the fetus: the social impact of amniocentesis in America*, London: Routledge.

Robertson, A.J. (1989) 'Histopathological grading of cervical intraepithelial neoplasia (CIN) – is there a need for change?', *Journal of Pathology*, 159: 273–5.

Royal National Board of Health (1966) *Gynaecological health investigation for early detection of cervical cancer* [Medicinalstyrelsen. Gynekologisk hälsoundersökning för tidig upptäckt av livmoderhalscancer], Nr 111. AB Nordiska Bokhandeln.

Ryle, J.A. (1961) 'The meaning of the normal', in Lush, B. (ed.) *Concepts of medicine: a collection of essays on aspects of medicine*, Oxford: Pergamon.

Singer, C. and Underwood, E.A. (1962) 'The rebirth of science', in *A short history of medicine*, Oxford: Clarendon Press.

Singleton, V. (1998a) 'Feminism, sociology of scientific knowledge and postmodernism: politics, theory and me', *Social Studies of Science*, 26: 445–68.

Singleton, V. (1998b) 'Stabilizing instabilities: the role of the laboratory in the United Kingdom cervical screening programme', in Berg, M. and Mol, A. (eds) *Differences in medicine: unraveling practices, techniques and bodies*, London: Duke University Press.

Star, S.L. and Griesemer, J.R. (1989) 'Institutional ecology, "translations" and boundary objects: amateurs and professionals in Berkeley's Museum of Vertebrate Zoology, 1907–39', *Social Studies of Science*, 19: 387–420.

Swedish Council on Technology Assessment in Health Care (SBU) (1996) 'Screening as technology', in 'Mass screening for prostate cancer', *International Journal of Cancer*, Suppl. 9: 13–17.

Swedish National Board of Health and Welfare (1998) *Gynaecological smear control: proposition for a screening program* [Socialstyrelsen, Gynekologisk cellprovskontroll. Förslag till screeningprogram], SoS-rapport 1998: 15.

Symonds, R.P. (1997) 'Screening for cervical cancer: different problems in the developing and the developed world', *European Journal of Cancer Care*, 6: 275–9.

The Report of the Cervical Cancer Inquiry (1988) Government Printing Office, Auckland.

Traweek, S. (1988) *Beamtimes and lifetimes: the world of high energy physicists*, Cambridge, MA: Harvard University Press.

Wied, G.L. (1964) 'Editorial. Pap-test or Babes method?', *Acta Cytologica*, 8: 173–4.

4 Gynaecologists and geneticists as storytellers

Disease, choice and normality as the fabric of narratives on pre-implantation genetic diagnosis

Kristin Zeiler

Introduction

During the past three decades, several technologies have been developed that allow medical professionals to assess the physical status of the foetus during a woman's pregnancy. On the one hand, it has been argued that use of these technologies can be reassuring for parents who worry that their child may have a certain genetic disease. They can receive knowledge on which to base decisions of whether to carry the pregnancy to term. It has also been argued that those who know that they are at risk of a certain genetic disease and who, therefore, dare not try for pregnancy may dare to do so thanks to the availability of these technologies. On the other hand, uses of the technologies have also been criticised for imposing psychological burdens (Hildt 2002), particularly on women (Lippman 1998). Today, technologies are not only available for assessment of the prenatal physical status of the foetus but also for the genetic diagnosis of the embryo.

Pre-implantation genetic diagnosis, hereafter referred to as PGD, implies a genetic testing of embryos, performed after an ex-corporeal assisted reproductive technology. Its aim is to identify the presence of genes that will or might result in a particular genetic disease, and it allows selective transfer and implantation of embryos into a woman's uterus. PGD can be offered to couples who know that they are at risk for a certain genetic disease. Furthermore, pre-implantation genetic *screening* of embryos can be offered to couples who undergo an ex-corporeal assisted reproductive technology but who are not at risk for a known genetic disease. The main aim of such genetic screening of embryos is to enhance the success-rate of the assisted reproductive technology, particularly for women above a certain age and women who have had previous miscarriages. These women's embryos may carry chromosomal deviations and such deviations have been considered a main reason why implantations fail or the women miscarry. Embryos with chromosomal deviations can be sorted out after genetic screening (Rubio *et al.* 2003).

The availability and use of assisted reproductive technologies combined with PGD evoke moral, social and existential questions. When PGD is discussed among health professionals and scientists, a number of stories are also told in which interpretations of disease, choice and normality are combined and re-combined in different ways. Some such narratives and some such interpretations will be explored in this chapter, which draws on the results of a project on moral aspects of pre-implantation genetic diagnosis in which 18 British, Italian and Swedish geneticists and gynaecologists have been interviewed.[1] The interviewees were chosen with the purpose of enabling a wide spectrum of reflections from within the medical profession. Such a spectrum was considered as enabled if geneticists and gynaecologists who worked at PGD units, in other (non-PGD) clinics as well as/or in research units were invited. Ten of the interviewees were women, eight were men.[2]

The choice of nationalities was based on the assumption that the different national legal approaches and policies toward PGD could enable a wide spectrum of reflections – again – from within the medical profession. The UK has more flexible guidelines with regard to PGD than Sweden. It is to be noted that in the UK, PGD has been used for genetic conditions such as familial adenomatous polyposis coli, which can lead to colon cancer in early adulthood.[3] According to HFEA's critics, this is a disease that usually appears in adult life and which is treatable (Bosch 2004; The Lancet 2004). Furthermore, the UK Human Fertilisation and Embryology Authority, hereafter referred to as HFEA, has given licence for PGD tissue typing that allows the selection of embryos in order to bring about the birth of a child who can provide a matched tissue donation for an existing sibling (HFEA 2001) – as well as for pre-implantation genetic screening for an 'abnormal' number of chromosomes. As regards Sweden, the policy has been to allow PGD only for the diagnosis of 'severe, progressive, hereditary diseases that lead to an early death' and where 'no cure or treatment' is available (SOU 1994/5 18:13). As an example, which also clarifies the difference between the UK and Sweden, the genetic condition of familial adenomatous polyposis coli (above) would not fulfil these criteria. However, the Swedish guidelines have been criticised (SMER 2004) and it has now been suggested that the last requirement should be dropped. PGD should be allowed to be used for severe, progressive chromosomal or structural genetic diseases (SOU 2004: 300–1).

As regards pre-implantation genetic screening, it has been suggested that it should not be used as a matter of routine but it should be allowed within distinct research projects that had been approved by a research ethical council (SOU 2004: 300). As a contrast to the UK and Sweden, Italy has had neither policy guidelines nor national bodies that regulate PGD clinics. It has been the most unregulated country of the three – and was the most unregulated country at the time of the interviews. Since 2004, Italy has had one of the strictest regulations, according to which all embryos that result after assisted reproductive technologies must be implanted (*Legge 19 Feb 2004 n.40, Norme in Materia di Procreazione Assistita*).

However, it is to be noted that the UK PGD clinics are regulated in a different sense the Swedish PGD clinics. In the UK, if a certain couple would like to use PGD for a genetic condition for which the PGD clinic in question has not been licensed to offer it, it is the professionals at the PGD unit who apply for such a licence at the Human Fertilisation and Embryology Authority. In Sweden, Socialstyrelsen (the National Board of Health and Welfare) must report all uses of PGD, but there is no licence system. In Italy, at the time of the interviews, no national licensing board existed (and since 2004 Italian law makes PGD pointless since all fertilised embryos must be implanted).

In the interviews with the 18 professionals, three major types of stories or narratives recurred. These narratives will be presented and discussed in this chapter. First, there were *narratives of life with genetic disease.* Most of these narratives resulted in descriptions of life with genetic disease as problematic and painful. Some of them indicated that though life with genetic disease could be tragic, there was also hope for couples concerned. Second, there were *narratives of progress* in terms of in different senses 'better' technologies being developed. These narratives resulted in descriptions of a technical progression underway that had positive psychological, moral and/or existential implications for future parents. Third, there were *narratives of concern*, which highlighted professionals' own concerns as regards how to describe, interpret and evaluate use of PGD.

Interpretations of disease, normality and choice were components of the fabric of the narratives, to a varying extent, and they were used in the construction of a certain logic – as well as in the questioning of this logic – within and throughout the different narratives.

The technologies: assisted reproductive technology and PGD

Pre-implantation genetic diagnosis presupposes that a woman and a man have used some kind of assisted reproductive technology. Some assisted reproductive technologies are performed in a woman's body (corporeal assisted reproductive) and some outside of her body (ex-corporeal assisted reproductive). It is only ex-corporeal assisted reproductive that is combined with PGD. One of the most common technologies for ex-corporeal assisted reproduction is *in vitro* fertilisation (*in vitro* meaning that it is performed outside the body, literally in glass).

In vitro fertilisation involves ovarian stimulation in order to cause a woman to produce extra oocytes. If present, oocytes are retrieved and placed in a culture medium that allows them to mature further. Mature eggs are put in a Petri dish with sperm and if fertilisation occurs, embryos are returned to the culture medium for further development. In some cases, eggs are instead fertilised by means of intracytoplasmic sperm injection. This involves injection of a single sperm into an egg with a glass needle and use of technology for micro-manipulating single cells and embryos without destroying them (technology for holding an unfertilised egg with a pipette while injecting the sperm).

PGD involves analysing one or two cells obtained from a six to ten cell-stage embryo – a stage reached three days after insemination.[4] Embryos are cultivated *in vitro* and a biopsy of one or two cells is taken from the embryo. A genetic analysis is performed on these cells, which allows transfer and implantation of embryos without the specific genetic disease. In some cases, this analysis can be performed by means of fluorescent marking of chromosomes or parts of chromosomes (fluorescent *in situ* hybridisation). Fluorescent *in situ* hybridisation implies that biomedical substances are used in order to make certain segments of chromosomes shine when exposed to ultra-violet light. It can be used to indicate sex as well as certain structural and numerical changes in the chromosomes. In the case of single-gene disease (and as it is not possible to detect a mutation in the DNA from a single cell without amplifying the relevant DNA sequence) all single-gene genetic analyses rely on single-cell polymerase chain reaction for such amplification (Braude *et al.* 2002). Polymerase chain reaction is used to amplify DNA to indicate single-gene diseases either when a certain DNA sequence mutation is identified or in linkage analysis when such a mutation is statistically linked to some other identifiable DNA sequence.

There are difficulties with all the alternatives and the risk of error due to the human factor is always present. Consequently, there are recommendations that PGD, if resulting in a pregnancy, shall be combined with prenatal diagnosis (SMER 2004:6) or, at least, that such combination shall be discussed with the woman and man concerned (Thornhill *et al.* 2005).

Narrative analysis

I use narrative analysis as a method for exploring ethically relevant phenomena that interviewees constructed and discussed in the form of narratives. I understand a narrative as a story of a sequence of events, which is significant for the person telling it. It has a plot and an internal logic that makes sense to the narrator (Denzin 1989). I consider the narrative to be something more than structural features of a text. A narrative is embedded in human action and the social context in which it is related as well as the narrator's reason for telling it are important elements in the understanding of it (Herrenstein-Smith 1981). I also concur with narrative researchers who hold that we, by using the narrative form, assign meaning to events, place events within a certain order and invest them with significance – and often with a moral significance (Whyte 1981; Polyani 1989).

A number of narrative styles and analytic distinctions applied to these styles are available and I have combined elements of different narrative analyses. I have identified *orientations*, which answers the questions of 'Who? What? When? Where?', *complications* which answers the question of 'then what happened?' and *evaluations* which answers the question 'so what?' (Labov 1972; Cortazzi 1993). In this sense, I draw on the work of those who elaborate narrative analysis with a concern for formal structural properties in relation to their function, but I do so with the purpose of exploring the narratives' *moral* or *point* (Polanyi 1989). Stories with a moral or a point have a long tradition and they are told with a certain purpose; a number of different morals/points can also be identified within a narrative (ibid.). I focus on the overall moral of the story, articulated when the interviewee explained how the events told shall be understood, explained and/or valued. This overall moral was often expressed in the narrative's evaluation. In this sense, the interviewed gynaecologists and geneticists became 'story-tellers' (Ettorre 1999).

Three types of narratives

Narratives of life with genetic disease

Within 'narratives of life with genetic disease', interviewees told stories of patients they had encountered, of members in their own families or, on a few occasions, their own personal experiences of life with genetic disease. Some of these narratives contained words such as tragedy or similar value-laden notions. Professionally, at the PGD clinic, Andrew said, he met with tragedy. But personally, it was different:

> I wouldn't want to have affected children, I certainly wouldn't. I wouldn't want to have a child who spends a great deal of its life, and it might be a shortened life or [a life] in contact with hospitals, always having uncomfortable or painful procedures, being unwell, being unable to keep up with the others at the same age, different schooling, anything like that. I couldn't bear to watch my own child have to struggle the whole way through its life and then probably lose it.

Andrew had relatives who had lost their child at an early age. Losing one's child, he said, was 'just the worst scenario'. Living with a severe genetic disease was sometimes described as a 'suffering' and living with a child with a severe genetic disease was sometimes described as 'distressing'; the death of a loved one was described as devastating.

Interviewees also articulated frustration and the wish to alter the situation for the couples concerned in a slightly different story-line within this type of narrative. These were stories that indicated that life with a genetic disease could be or was painful, but the stories ended with descriptions of a situation where some diseases could be avoided or were avoided. The potential tragedy and pain was spoken of as being able to be minimised through use of assisted reproductive technologies and PGD, for those to whom these technologies were available, and who wanted them. These couples could choose to try to avoid a(nother) child with a genetic disease. Descriptions of the possible value of disease prevention through selection of embryos were always conditioned: emphasis was put on the value of being able to prevent disease if the couple concerned so wished, and *not* disease prevention as such.

The primary focus of these narratives was directed at the experiences of grown-up women and men who either had a particular genetic disease, were carriers of a genetic disease or who worried that they or their partner could be a carrier. This focus also harmonises with the description of hope as a matter of choice for parents. Grown-up women and men were described as experiencing or considering life with a certain genetic disease as painful, as being in need of medical help or as asking for medical technologies that would help them to avoid a(nother) child with the particular disease.

In the evaluation of these narratives, some interviewees also explained that it was understandable if certain couples wanted to avoid the birth of a child with a particular disease. 'Naturally' we want our future child to be healthy. Who would not want to do so, Simonetta remarked. Through such statements, interviewees not only described their views on couples' use of PGD, they also legitimatised couples' use of PGD. Life with genetic disease could be tragic, it could be avoided, and who would not like a healthy child? One interviewee also said that though one should have respect for those who were handicapped in different ways, being handicapped 'was no merit'.

Simonetta not only explained that it was natural to want healthy children, she also described healthy children as normal children. This was the case when she commented on the hypothetical story of a mother with two previous children with a genetic disease who wanted to use PGD for a third child, wondering that though it was 'ugly' to say so, was there not a 'right to a small slice of normality'? In this context, the normal is to have children without a certain genetic disease. Her statement that it was ugly to say so indicated an awareness that this view may be controversial. Still, she described the wish to have healthy/normal children as natural.[5]

If the story-line of narratives of life with genetic disease is to be summarised, there were certain threads that were common to most of these stories, such as the descriptions of tragedy and pain, of the frustration on behalf of the interviewees if there was nothing they could do, of the wish to avoid genetic disease in one's children if possible and, in some narratives, of hope in terms of the possibility, for some women and men, to choose to use PGD and to implant embryos without the particular disease. It is also to be noted that there were a few narratives of life with genetic disease that neither focused on tragedy nor on hope in terms of the possibility to use PGD. These narratives were told by the interviewee who had personal, embodied[6] experience of genetic disease and this interviewee emphasised how grateful he was to live.

Narratives of progress

Narratives of progress indicated that there was an on-going technical progression within medicine. Technologies had been or were being developed which were, in different senses, described as better than previous technologies. PGD was described as a psychologically and/or morally easier means to avoid the birth of a child with a genetic disorder than prenatal diagnosis and selective termination of pregnancy. It was described as technically better than technologies for genetic diagnosis of foetuses. It was also described as positive since it meant that some couples were given choice and the possibility of (some) reproductive control, *independently* of whether PGD resulted in the birth of a healthy child. There was something to offer to patients and this was described as positive also for the interviewees themselves as professionals. When taken together, narratives of life with genetic disease and narratives of progress resulted in a certain logic. There were couples who faced tragic situations (couples who had a 'genuine need' for PGD as one of the British interviewees phrased it) and medical professionals could help some of those in need through the provision of a new, important and helpful diagnostic method.

Interviewees described the difference between (different) previous and present situations in detail. As a general tendency, previous situations, situations where there was no diagnostic method available or the early prenatal diagnosis situation, were depicted as difficult, terrible and in different senses undesirable whereas the present situation, the PGD-situation, was better (though not unproblematic). When this contrast was given, focus was directed at the technical progress and the positive consequences of this progress.

In the early prenatal diagnosis situation, in the 1950s, some interviewees explained, there were no choices.[7] Others said that there were choices but that these were painful. These situations were 'horrific' in Joyce's vocabulary. Joyce explained that some women did not dare to become pregnant since they suspected that they were carriers of a genetic disease. Others, who expected either themselves or their partners to be carriers of a severe x-bound genetic disease, would terminate any male pregnancy in order to escape the risk of giving birth to a severely sick son. Daughters were born, this interviewee recalled, since they would either be non-affected or be carriers. Joyce also told the story of some of the women she met in counselling, who had only 10 per cent or 20 per cent risk of being carriers of a particular genetic disease. 'You knew,' she said, 'and they knew, that the baby that they'd aborted was probably normal. They just couldn't take that chance and that was awful, I mean, it was so tragic for them'. In the narrative's evaluation, Ann concluded that 'sometimes' she 'wanted to scream at them, take your chances, it might be all right. But of course, you cannot say such things'.

Different kinds of prenatal diagnoses represented the first steps in the stair of progression; more and more accurate kinds of methods were described as being developed, which allowed the women concerned to plan future pregnancies to an extent that had not been possible before. As narratives of progress unfolded, further progress was described as expected.

Joyce's narrative of progress did not encompass PGD as a clear matter of progress, but other interviewees did. The availability of PGD was described as having positive consequences for women and men at high risk for genetic diseases. There was a technology that could meet the needs of those couples. It was also, sometimes, described as having positive consequences for medical professionals in their everyday work. Such was the case when Åsa explained that for some women and men, who may have gone through PND (prenatal diagnosis) and abortion or miscarried several times, PGD was a 'last straw to clutch at' and she concluded that 'it always feels good to have been able to offer something more [to these couples]'. Such was also the case when Andrew explained that the possibility of PGD made his everyday work 'easier' even if it did not always result in the birth of a healthy child.

Let us take a closer look at Andrew's narrative of progress. It started with an orientation, where the pre-PGD situation was described as 'frustrating' and as offering little possibility of acting. There was little or nothing 'to offer'. In his words:

> I would meet somebody with translocation who had recurrent miscarriages. In the cases of translocations, it used to be, it would be very frustrating. I would see somebody with recurrent miscarriages who had a translocation or a husband with a translocation. You couldn't do anything other than roll the dice each time. Maybe you'd get lucky. Whereas now you can actually offer something concrete.

The metaphor 'roll the dice' is noteworthy. The rolling of the dice, used by the Romans in order to find out what destiny, fate or chance had in store, was used as a means to describe the conditions of hazard that couples had to live under – conditions that doctors could not change. Before PGD and particularly before prenatal diagnosis and molecular diagnosis, rolling the dice was a necessity because of the absence of alternatives: couples who knew that they were at risk for a particular disease had to choose between not becoming parents and accepting that the child born might have a serious disease (or, when adoption was available, adopting). This was no longer the case – rolling the dice was no longer necessary – though PGD was still no certain way to children without a particular genetic disease.

Andrew's narrative continued with him explaining that before he started to work at the PGD clinic, he had not reflected on the situations of some of the couples that he now met every day. Meeting them was an 'eye-opener'.

> They were always in genetics, but it hadn't crossed my mind that they existed, to be honest. It was a real eye-opener to see them. I think it must have been really difficult to have been a geneticist before PGD was available, to see couples with these awful conditions and not be able to offer anything at all. At least for some of them, now there's something to offer. It doesn't always help but at least there's something else for them, if they want it.

The introduction of PGD is the peak and the turning-point of this narrative, present in the narrative's complication. Before PGD was available, there was nothing to offer and this lack of options, Andrew stated, must have made the work 'really difficult'. In the narrative's evaluation, this interviewee concluded that 'at least for some of them, now there's something to offer'. In Andrew's view, this was positive – even if PGD did not always help. Technical progression was positive *even* if it did not result in the birth of a healthy, biological child. It provided certain couples with more or better alternatives to choose between. In a similar focus on choice as the positive consequence of the availability of PGD, Joyce explained that PGD was valuable if couples received a healthy child but that it was 'more important' that couples were given a choice. She explained that 'usually most people's desired outcome is the birth of a healthy child but what's more important to me, I think, is the fact that people are given a choice'.

Narratives of concern

The logic derived from narratives of life with genetic disease and narratives of progress – that life with genetic disease could be tragic, that some couples had a medical problem that needed to be met, that PGD meant progress and that it was a means to meet the medical need – was questioned in narratives of concern. Within this category of narratives, interviewees told stories of risks related to the offer or use of IVF/PGD, such as the risk of physical pain and psychological distress due to the treatments, risk of misdiagnosis or risks that couples were not given accurate information of the treatments. Interviewees also told stories of actual, complicating circumstances (that was not a matter of risks) such as in the story of a woman and man who used IVF and PGD in order to test for and avoid a particular genetic disease in their offspring, but the child born had another disease which had not been tested for and the woman and man had not realised that this could be the case. Finally, interviewees told stories of exaggerated uses and misuses of the technology, present and future, such as the story in which professionals offered PGD for what they later considered conditions for which PGD should not have been used, typically expressed by one interviewee who said that 'we got caught up in the enthusiasm of PGD actually working, it seemed fine at that time. But it isn't fine, really'.

These narratives resulted in interviewees' concern of how to describe and evaluate use of the technology. As a first example of a narrative of concern, concern was the result of the perceived risk that women and men did not get accurate information about PGD or about alternatives to PGD.

Joyce was one of the interviewees who told her personal story of IVF experiences. She also described her frustration with how IVF and PGD were presented in British media and she told stories of risks that couples were given inaccurate information. In her view, what had happened was that

> people have been sold the good news stories. It's been a lot of television programs on this, and it's often been wrongly portrayed as the only way that a couple can have a healthy baby when faced with a genetic risk.

Joyce was concerned about the way PGD was presented and described and she held that women and men did not necessarily get accurate information – they were sold the good news stories – and there were other stories as well, which needed to be told. 'It affects me,' she said, because she wondered whether doctors 'had explained to them the other option' of prenatal diagnosis and an early termination of pregnancy, and 'whether both options were spelled out to them in an equal way'. Joyce also explained that she was 'not anti-PGD', but that she felt that 'there's quite a lot of zealots around who are so pro it, that they sometimes minimize the down-side of it and ignore other options'.

The reason for caution was lack of information and biased information and this lack or bias also resulted in concern as well as ambivalence on behalf of Joyce of how to evaluate PGD. On the one hand, PGD could be positive for some. On the other hand, PGD had been sold as a good news story, to an extent that was not correct.

Other interviewees commented on the structures in which PGD was offered as well as on how they as medical professionals discussed PGD with couples. In these narratives of concern, interviewees described actual, complicating circumstances that rendered the clinical encounter difficult. This was the case when Andrew told the stories of some couples that he met in clinic. In his words:

> I've become more and more worried that, if a couple want treatment, we feel obliged to offer it to them [and it is] not always in their best interest, but simply because they want it and we can do it. Then, we are almost supporting them, pushing them towards it. Of course, they're going to be, if they want something they're going to be very vocal about it, because they have to have been quite vocal and persistent to have got as far as us. So they're never going to say to the doctor 'I think I want to have this'. You know, they might not turn up for treatment, but they are going to have to say 'We really want this, we must have this now', and so then we end up saying 'Yes, you must have it now'. Before you know it, we've done the treatment. We'll, we never stepped back to say, you know, 'Just because they wanted it, was it the right thing to do for that individual?'

In this excerpt, Andrew described himself as contributing to the pressure on couples concerned: he pushed them.[8] The excerpt also contained the idea of a vicious circle, where one part pushed the other and vice versa. Medical professionals pushed couples, couples needed to be persistent, the more persistent they sounded, the more professionals felt that couples should use the technology and be offered it etc. Andrew expressed concern about the consequences of this vicious circle. Little space was left to encourage reflections, articulations of doubts and hesitance. If present, he continued, such reflections were seldom articulated but shown through possible absences during treatment – couples did not show up later, when expected. This was undesirable and it worried him.

Andrew described how he and his colleagues pushed couples in a certain direction, but it is also interesting to note that some interviewees (Andrew included) described situations in which *they* felt pushed by couples to offer PGD for conditions for which they did not want to offer it. Interviewees also told stories and described situations in which they wondered if other patient groups did not push couples in a certain direction (and to an undesirable extent). Again, these narratives focused on circumstances of the clinical encounter that made things complicated. What took place in the clinical encounter was not what interviewees wanted to take place. Furthermore, these narratives highlighted the socio-cultural context in which the choice to try PGD as well as the use of PGD took place. As one example, this was the case when Andrew described support networks for couples at risk of a certain genetic disease, where groups of people who wanted to use PGD were described as questioning those who did not. In this reflection, Andrew related the issue of choice to guilt. He framed it as a question, addressed by those who did want to use PGD. If those who do not want to use PGD have children, he said, some of these children will be affected and die. How do those who use PGD view these couples? Do they blame them for having chosen to give birth to these children?

> I wonder how couples who have only had unaffected children because they've terminated the affected or only have unaffected children because they've had a successful PGD view those families. I suspect they probably think that those couples have no right to have an affected child.

Here, certain couples at risk for genetic diseases, who had or wanted to use PGD, were ascribed the role of those who questioned couples who did not want to use PGD, but Andrew also reflected on his own view and his own understanding of who should use PGD. In his words, 'It's very insidious, I even find myself thinking now "they don't have a right to have that", but of course, they have a right to have an affected child'.

As another example of stories of actual, complicating circumstances, a few interviewees described the situation in which to decide whether to use PGD as so complex and so filled with morally delicate questions, that they wondered if it was desirable to keep to the ideal of non-advice discussions in the genetic counselling. Again, an excerpt from the interview with Andrew will be presented. Andrew exemplified his reasoning with a story of a couple that he had encountered:

> I remember one couple very clearly. They said, you know, they never wanted to know about this kind of thing, but it's not choice, there's not a choice [...] Couples come to see me who might have no educational background, you know, he might be a window cleaner and she might be a housewife. Suddenly, they have to think about numbers of embryos [...] morphology of embryos that was way beyond what they normally

expected to confront in their lives, and they're faced with ethical questions that in many ways they're really unprepared to be able to face. I think they become swamped by it sometimes. Suddenly they have to think within a very short time-scale as well.

In this interviewee's view, PGD evoked more moral questions than most people met during a lifetime and this during a restricted period. The risk of information overload was present, in the sense that too much information was given and that information also meant that a number of complex moral issues had to be addressed. Furthermore (as seen in the beginning of the excerpt), being informed about PGD was not a choice. This was problematic, couples could no longer choose not to choose, even though they might wish to. This idea was articulated in a particularly clear way by another interviewee, Alva. Information forced couples into a situation of choice in which they had to face questions such as should they listen to the information, how should they judge the information and should they base their decisions on it? In Alva's view, 'the problem' of choosing PGD was 'that you do not choose information'. 'It sounds as if we inform very innocently and most people ask for information', she reflected, 'but there are people who wished that they had not needed to choose'. Information given precluded the possibility of choosing not to know and not to choose and in this sense it conveyed restrictions on what couples could and would choose.

Finally, there were narratives that highlighted interviewees' own uncertainty concerning how to interpret others' experiences of life with genetic disease. This first uncertainty was often related to a second one: the uncertainty of whether there were any non-subjective definitions of genetic disease that could be used in the discussion of what diseases to search for with PGD. These stories highlighted actual, complicating aspects of the offer of PGD. How should it be described and for which genetic diseases should it be offered?

Simonetta was one of the interviewees who told a story that highlighted both of the above-described uncertainties. She told the life story of Michel Petrucciani, a jazz musician with a rare genetic disease that made his bones break continually, with resulting malformations. Petrucciani, Simonetta said, was not more than one metre tall and he had serious health problems. He died because of a respiration crisis. Still, she said, 'he had chosen to give birth to a male child, affected as he was. [...] I don't want a child with his disease, I don't, but he existed and he has done great things'.

Throughout this narrative, Simonetta clarified difficulties in assessing life with genetic disease. In the narrative's evaluation, she explained that she would not like to have a child with the disease, but that Petrucciani, who had that experience, did. She also explained that the story of Petrucciani made her question the possibility to elaborate an objective definition of disease; the reason she gave was that the severity of a disease could not be assessed by anyone except the person who had the disease.

The emphasis on the perspective and the experiences of the person living with the disease was present in most interviews, but in two slightly different versions. Sometimes, interviewees emphasised the importance of what I call *lived experiences*. Such experiences included personal experiences of close relatives with a genetic disease (whom someone lived with/had lived with) as well as personal experiences of having a particular genetic disease. Sometimes, interviewees only referred to the latter sub-category of lived experiences, the *embodied experiences*, i.e. personal experiences of a genetic disease that someone has, in her or his own physical body. A few interviewees also told narratives that indicated that they doubted that anyone could be able to – and should – decide what disease might be tragic and painful to live with except the (future) person with that disease.

The narratives of concern described here resulted in six different concerns or worries. As seen in the narratives of life with genetic disease and narratives of progress and as will be discussed in the next section of this chapter, the availability of informed choice was a main issue and a reason why PGD was described as positive. Within the narratives of concern much of the concerns/worries were related to choice – but also to genetic disease. First, within these narratives, interviewees held choice to be important, but they worried that choice was *not as informed and free as they thought it should be*. Second, they worried that there *was no or little possibility to choose*. Third, they worried that they, as professionals, were pushed in certain directions and that *patient groups infringed their own choices*. Fourth, they worried that patients would *ask for PGD for* what they considered as *undesirable uses*. Fifth, they worried that the *choice was too complicated* for (some) couples and this made them question the idea of non-advice genetic counselling with regard to use of PGD. Sixth and finally, they were concerned about their own *inability to understand* life with genetic disease and the difficulty to find non-subjective definitions of genetic disease.

Underpinnings of the narratives: exploring the fabric

In what senses were disease, normality and choice the fabric of the narratives? In narratives of life with genetic disease, life with genetic disease was described as tragic and painful. Tragedies were described as difficult to avoid and particularly so for couples with genetic diseases that could not be tested for with PGD. Within these narratives, choice was mainly commented upon in subordinated clauses. Couples were described as having no choice or having few alternatives to choose between. There were also narratives in which life with genetic disease was described as tragic and painful, but in these narratives there was also a means to avoid the tragedies in terms of the birth of future children with genetic disease. There was hope for those in need and this hope was primarily framed in the language of choice. Some couples were given choice and, if so, this was positive.

It is noteworthy that it was the possibility to try to avoid genetic disease, if one so wanted, that was described as important, not disease avoidance as such. Choice resulted as more important than disease avoidance, even if choice was positive as a possible means to disease avoidance. Still, the logic within these narratives was underpinned by the idea that life with genetic disease could be tragic and painful (compare Shakespeare 1999: 672–5; 2003).[9] These descriptions also harmonise with certain aspects of what some call 'the medical model' in disability theory: the tragedy of the individual was emphasised (as opposed to an emphasis on the failure of a society that disables some people) (Reindal 2000: 89).[10]

The emphasis on tragedy and pain in these narratives of life with genetic disease also, sometimes, resulted in two different uses of normality. First, the notion of normality was used to make a certain wish legitimate: it was nothing strange to want to avoid genetic disease in future children. It was a normal/natural wish that most of us would share. Second, healthy children were also, sometimes, described as the normal ones. In the latter descriptions, some interviewees used what some philosophers have labelled a 'naive non-scientific usage' of the notion of normality in medicine: health was associated with normality, disease with abnormality and health meant absence of disease (Hoedemaekers and ten Have 1999: 539–40).[11] Though this understanding of normality can be used in order to indicate that normality – i.e. health – is desirable, it is important to note that it is not necessarily so.

The normality of healthy children and the description of the normality of wanting to have normal/healthy children begs for further reflection. 'Lurking in all genetic theory and practice is the disturbing question of the "normal"', says feminist theologian Karen Lebacqz. In her view, this question is disturbing if or when the normal is the basis for a norm of standard for what we should be like and if those who do not fit the norm are presumed to be 'inferior, inadequate, in need of therapy' (1999: 89–90). So it would be particularly disturbing, others explain, if the normal is associated with the establishment of genetic norms (Wolf 1995: 345–53). Whereas this disturbing question has been focused upon in the literature, only three interviewees commented upon it, and they did so when they told stories of future undesirable scenarios of 'designer babies' and alleged 'perfect' societies in which selection had gone too far (perfection in this story-line was not an ideal but a threat) – i.e. in narratives of concern of misuses.[12] PGD was only questioned on the basis that it presumed an undesirable genetic norm in three interviews.

The description of the normal wish to have normal/healthy children can also evoke the question of what is not normal, what wishes or behaviours do not qualify as normal? If it is normal to want to have normal children, having 'non-normal' children when it could be avoided could be regarded as 'non-normal' or 'abnormal'. However, this view was *not* articulated by the interviewees.[13] Within narratives of life with genetic disease, it is also noteworthy that it was not the desire to choose that was described as normal, but the desire to avoid genetic disease.

Choice, genetic disease and normality were threads in narratives of progress as well. PGD was described as more accurate than previous technologies, less psychologically painful and morally easier (for some). Furthermore, PGD was described as a matter of positive progress since it meant that some couples were given one more choice. Some couples, who had not considered previous alternatives as realistic options for them, were given choice and choice was described as positive if it resulted in the birth of a child without a particular genetic disease. Choice was *also* described as positive as such (as in the excerpt 'it does not always help but at least there's something else for them'), independently of whether it resulted in the birth of a healthy child. As was the case in narratives of genetic disease, avoidance of genetic disease was never explicitly described as positive as such.[14]

The value of choice and disease avoidance (sometimes phrased as disease prevention) recur in descriptions of genetic counselling in bioethical literature. Genetic counselling, some suggest, 'does not aim to prevent couples from having children with genetic diseases. Preventing genetic disorders, although important, is secondary to good clinical practice, which identifies couples at risk and by empathic counselling allows them to make their own informed choice' (Harris 1998: 335). As remarked by Lene Koch and Mette Nordahl-Svendsen (2005), this presentation results in a distinction between the goals of disease prevention and informed choice; informed choice is described as primary to disease prevention.[15] The results of the analysis of my empirical data concur with this emphasis on informed choice. Within narratives of progress, provision of choice is described as primary to disease avoidance, from the medical professionals' point of view. Here it is also to be noted that there may be a discrepancy between what patients consider as the important outcome of PGD, what medical professionals consider as important and what medical professionals believed patients consider important (such as in Joyce's remark that she thought patients' desired outcome was the birth of a healthy child whereas she thought it was more important that patients were given choice).

Narratives of progress showed that provision of choice was described as positive for professionals. It made their work 'easier'. How can this be understood? In one reading, which takes medical professional identity as a point of departure, medical professionals are trained to treat/alleviate disease or promote health. They find themselves in a situation where people ask for help, where professionals are unable to treat the disease, but where they can, at least, provide couples with one more choice. Being able to provide couples with another choice can make it psychologically easier for professionals to work than if no choices or treatments could be provided.

In their discussion of genetic counselling, Koch and Nordahl-Svendsen (2005) suggest that problems need not only make people look for solutions. Solutions also provide a framework for statement and handling of certain problems. If applied to the PGD context and situations of some genetic diseases for which PGD is offered, there is no treatment. There is a technology that can be used to sort out embryos with some genetic diseases, but obviously this is not treatment in the ordinary sense. If PGD is a solution to these situations, it is a solution in terms of choice and not treatment. This can also be a reason why some professionals suggest that choice is more important than disease avoidance.[16]

Within narratives of progress, the thread of normality entered the narratives in the form of comments as in phrases 'the baby being born, that they'd aborted, was probably normal'. When this was done, normality was used in order to indicate that the child had not had the particular disease that parents wanted to avoid. However, if normality is linked to health as was sometimes done by the interviewees, this can result in images of 'normal' women and men (without 'genetic problems') as well as of 'normal patients' (families with a genetic problem) (Ettorre 1999: 544). This being the case, it is the 'normal patients' who are described as needing PGD.

Finally, narratives of concern implied a questioning of the logic derived from the other narratives – did PGD really mean progress, was life with genetic disease tragic, had these patients a need that medical professionals could meet in a desirable and positive way – and the questioning, they said, made them ambivalent in terms of how to describe and evaluate use of PGD. As seen, narratives of concern resulted in a number of concerns on behalf of the medical professionals and many of these concerns were related to choice. If, as I have said, PGD cannot be seen as a matter of treatment but only as a matter of provision of choice (one more alternative, a psychologically and morally better alternative for some), it is understandable that choice is given a crucial function in many of the narratives.

Choice was described as important in narratives in which interviewees said they wondered if couples 'really' could choose (there were hampering influences, which made choice difficult and lack of real choice was considered as a problem). A certain choice had also become non-optional when couples could no longer choose not to choose and this was seen as problematic and as a reason for hesitance.

Within some of the narratives of concern, genetic disease was a main thread. This was the case when interviewees told stories that made them question their own ability to understand and evaluate life with genetic disease. These narratives also made them question the very possibility for non-subjective definitions of genetic disease – and in the long run – whether definitions of genetic diseases could and/ or should guide the decision of what diseases to test for and which embryos to sort out. Interestingly, these concerns were, again, related to choice. Which embryos should be allowed to be sorted out – i.e. not chosen for implantation – and who should decide which embryos were allowed to be sorted out, for which genetic conditions? Who should decide if not those who were able to understand the situation for those women, men and children who lived with a particular genetic disease, i.e. these people themselves? At the same time, some interviewees were concerned that 'people' would like to use PGD for genetic conditions that they, as professionals, did not think was desirable.

Some narratives of concern also contained normality as a thread. This was the case in stories of future undesirable scenarios which interviewees described as worrying and as reasons for their concern and ambivalence. Normality was also present in some narratives of concern, in a different and not so explicit sense than the ones discussed so far. As seen, some of the narratives of concern focused on risks of different kinds, there were physical and psychological risks for women undergoing treatment and there were risks for misdiagnosis. Was there a 'risk' that different risks became normalised, in the sense of common and accepted parts of everyday clinical practice, i.e. risks that professionals were aware of, found undesirable and tried to make explicit to couples, but which still became a 'normal' part and parcel of the treatment? Whereas most interviewees told stories of risks, only one interviewee commented on the low success-rate and he was upset that so few people questioned the very use of the methods on this basis. (What other methods would be allowed, this interviewee asked, in which only 20 per cent of the treatments were successful in the sense that a healthy, biological child was born?)[17] Had risks become normal? Finally, it is worth noting that the normality of wanting to have healthy children through the means of PGD was seldom questioned or problematised.[18]

Discussion and concluding comments

The results of the analysis of the empirical data presented in this chapter point to some issues that need to be further analysed. Choice resulted as a major thread in the narratives. What does choice in the field of reproductive genetics mean and what should characterise a desirable situation of choice in genetic counselling? Elsewhere, I have argued that abilities and opportunities (i) to reflect on what really matters to the persons engaged in choice, with regard to their reproduction, (ii) to come to a decision and (iii) to act upon it are important *if* someone can be said to have an autonomous choice in this particular field. It is important to enhance both the abilities and possibilities of such choice (Zeiler 2005, see also Meyers 1989).[19]

However, it is also important to note that whereas choice and autonomous choice have been much discussed in bioethics (Beauchamp and Childress 2001; Faden and Beauchamp 1986), this focus has also been questioned (Dodds 2000). In what can be called a *twofold empirical criticism* in the discussion of autonomy, it is sometimes argued, on an empirical basis, that not everyone wants to choose (Schneider 1998)[20] and that those who want to do so, do not always manage to do so. In my data, I take the presence of hampering influences on conditions for choice and autonomous choice to indicate that choice and autonomous choice within reproductive genetics were not always present (see also Zeiler 2005; Corrigan 2003; Hildt 2002). Furthermore, it has been argued that the rhetoric of reproductive choice in fact prevents us from examining the context in which reproduction becomes institutionalised (Raymond 1995). There are, to say the least, many complexities of choice in medicine (Lupton 1997).

Choice in the PGD situation is also different from choice in many other medical settings. A comparison between situations of choice in medicine in general, with some exceptions, and situations of choice at the PGD clinic can clarify this point. In the case of medicine in general, there is most often one patient. Whereas this patient may choose to discuss her or his situation with others who s/he wants to discuss it with such as family, friends, other experts in the field, s/he need not do so. The patient can choose to keep the diagnosis to her- or himself. No matter if the patient discusses the situation with others, the diagnosis is relevant to the patient's health status and not the health status of others.[21] Even if s/he chooses to discuss what to do and whether to undergo treatment with others, these others are not involved in the same sense. Though the consequences of a patient's choice can be very significant for some others, such as partner and/or children, these others will not necessarily undergo treatment themselves. If the patient chooses to undergo surgery, the person treated for a disease is also the one who has the disease. All of these aspects of medicine in general are either not as straightforward or different in the new reproductive medicine. In the latter, when IVF and PGD are used, the 'patient' is not one person, but at least two persons who cannot or dare not conceive a child together without technical and medical means. Neither of the so-called patients needs to have a manifest disease, but one or both of them need to be carriers of a disease.[22] Also, if one or both of the patients have a manifest disease, and even though the disease is the reason why they approach the hospital, their disease will not be treated, nor necessarily will consequences of that disease be treated. Furthermore, both patients/partners need to be involved in the discussion of whether and to undergo treatment, and if so which.[23] In addition, the genetic knowledge that is obtained is of relevance not only for the patients but for also siblings and other relatives. In situations in which PGD is offered and used, there is as yet no treatment of the disease for the future child. There is no treatment or alleviation from disease, only selection of embryos on the basis of genetic information.

Whereas some of these conditions are common for the prenatal diagnosis situation as well, the choice in the PGD context has one obvious and special feature: when the discussion of whether to use PGD takes place there is no embryo, no pregnancy, no foetus, no child. Conception, *in vitro*, has not yet taken place. Though choice in general and autonomous choice in traditional medicine have their complexities, some of these complexities are sharpened in the PGD context. Here, choices typically involve at least two persons and these persons are engaged in the shared decision-making in a way that is different from that which is most often found in medicine in general.

PGD is not a matter of treatment, nor is a pregnancy underway. It is offered as a possibility to select embryos, if one so wants. This can be one key to understand interviewees' ambivalence in how to evaluate PGD as well as their emphasis on the value of providing choice. Whereas they could have described PGD as positive since genetic diseases could be avoided, disease avoidance through PGD and selective transfer of embryos (as well as through prenatal diagnosis and abortion) has been criticised by networks for people with genetic disease/disability. These methods, it has been held, make women and men with a genetic disease/disability feel undesired and unequal and this is ethically problematic (DHR 1998, 2001). Providing choice has *not* been criticised in this way.

Choice provision can be seen as an important element of the 'work-place ideology' in reproductive genetics (compare Bosk 1993). This leads to other questions. If treatment or alleviation of disease cannot be seen as the goal of PGD, should provision of choice qualify as a desirable and acceptable goal – not only of PGD – but of reproductive genetics? What kind of choices should be provided and why? What strategies can be developed to ensure that those who do not wish to choose to take a stand can be given this opportunity – at least as soon as the professionals realise the couples' wish? If this is not done, we need also to ask if we are *obliged* to understand and to enact our lives in terms of choice, at least in reproductive genetics?[24] Obviously, choices may or may not be positive, they may be morally complex and psychologically painful to the extent that we do not wish to choose.

It seems as if the very existence of PGD results in a situation that, in part, promotes something that is described as valuable, namely choice, and, in part, does not. If so, it is understandable that the existence of PGD evokes ambivalence.

The narratives that I have explored are only narratives told by medical professionals. The perspective of women and men undergoing PGD treatment has been analysed in an ethnographic study by Sarah Franklin and Celia Roberts. When the results of these studies are compared, two similarities emerge. First, in both projects, respondents emphasise that the use of PGD was not easy. Roberts and Franklin concluded that many patients were eager to distinguish the choice to use PGD from trivial '"consumer" or narcissistic' choices. Instead, the choice to use PGD was a 'choice out of necessity' (Roberts and Franklin 2004). In a related manner, several of my interviewees underlined that the choice to use PGD was by no means easy for couples. The description of assisted reproductive technologies and PGD as a 'last straw to clutch at', as one interviewee put it, also concurs with the description of 'last chance babies' in studies of the experiences and views of women undergoing IVF (Modell 1989; Franklin 1997).

However, if IVF or IVF and PGD should qualify as a last straw or a last chance, this implies either that what is discussed is only biological children or that (if present in a general discussion about having children) adoption is not an acceptable or possible alternative. Second, on the basis of an analysis of the many ways in which PGD 'patients' got to PGD clinics, the reasons why they did so, how they experienced the procedures involved in PGD and how they moved on from PGD, Franklin and Roberts (forthcoming) conclude that PGD seems to be a site of extreme ambivalence in terms of how to understand, describe and value the technology.

Acknowledgements

Special thanks to the anonymous interviewees in the project. I am also grateful to the Swedish ELSA-program who financed this project as a whole, to the Church of Sweden who financed the research stay in Italy during which

Italian interviews were performed and to STINT, the Swedish Foundation for International Cooperation in Research and Higher Education, who financed the research stay in the UK during which British interviews were performed.

Notes

1 An ELSA-funded research project on ethical aspects of pre-implantation genetic diagnosis and germ-line gene therapy. See Zeiler (2005).

2 The Swedish interviews were performed in Swedish, the British interviews in English and most of the Italian ones in Italian. Some of the Italian interviewees said that they spoke English very well and that they could speak English during the interview. If so, we chose English as the language for these interviews. All interviews were performed by me.

3 On 1 November 2004, the Human Fertilisation Embryology Authority, hereafter referred to as HFEA, confirmed that it had given permission for screening of familial adenomatous polyposis coli, which can lead to colon cancer in early adulthood.

4 Polar body biopsy is another method for PGD. It is performed before fertilisation of an embryo. However, since the examples in this chapter only discuss PGD on embryos, I will not describe the method for polar body biopsy here (see Zeiler 2005 for such a description).

5 Finally, some interviewees described infertility as a disease and as something that was not normal. Infertile couples were contrasted with the 'normal' population. This was the case when one interviewee explained that 'we' have understood 'IVF as infertile, as a handicapped group of people that we help' as opposed to the 'normal' population. If so, for people with fertility difficulties, using assisted reproductive technologies would make them resemble the normal population. They could, thanks to medicine, enhance their chances of receiving a biological child.

6 I use the term 'personal, embodied experience' for the professional who had experience of a particular genetic disease/disability in his own body, i.e. not only experience of relatives, siblings or children with the disease. The latter experience is of course personal, but not embodied in the sense I have in mind.

7 At this time, prenatal diagnosis was mostly used for diagnosis of Down's syndrome or for foetal sexing for genetic conditions such as Duchenne's muscular dystrophy, interviewees said.

8 PGD units in Britain and Sweden are centralised and only a few such units exist. This, interviewees explained, had consequences for what took place in the clinical encounters. Normally, when a couple wanted to use PGD and when the medical professionals at their local hospital considered this as appropriate, the professionals got in contact with the PGD unit and made sure that PGD was available for that specific condition. In practice, according to some of the interviewees, these structures (though important with regard to having national control over what was offered, under what circumstances, and by what means) resulted in couples needing to be very verbal and to sound as if they were convinced that they wanted PGD, in order to be sent to PGD centres in the first place.

9 In his review of medical discourse on disability in international medical journals, Tom Shakespeare identifies 'narratives of tragedy' and 'narratives of optimism' similar to the kinds of *narratives of life with genetic disease* that I have identified (Shakespeare 1999: 673–7).

10 It has also been suggested that this model should be called the '"harmed condition" model of disability' (Harris 2000: 99). As regards attitudes to genetic diseases, a 36-nation survey of 2,901 geneticists and genetic counsellors showed that, as a global tendency, many of the interviewees said they would emphasise negative aspects of genetic diseases, such as Down's syndrome or cystic fibrosis, so that couples 'will favour termination of pregnancy without suggesting it directly' (Wertz and Fletcher 1998: 499). Fifty-eight per cent of the 12 geneticist respondents in Sweden said they would 'emphasize negative aspects so they will favour termination of pregnancy without suggesting it directly' in the case of Down's syndrome and cystic fibrosis. Such would be the case for 50 per cent of the 22 Italian geneticist respondents with regard to Down's syndrome and for 38 per cent of them with regard to cystic fibrosis. Such was also the case for 15 per cent of the 102 British geneticist respondents with regard to Down's syndrome and for 10 per cent of them with regard to cystic fibrosis (Wertz and Fletcher 1998: 499). For another study of attitudes to genetic diseases, within four European countries, see also Marteau *et al.* (1994a, 1994b).

11 In scientific language, these authors claim, disease is either associated with the structure and function of the body or parts of the body or it is discussed in terms of multi-factorial contributive causes. Such a language was also present in the interviews, but not in relation to discussions of normality.

12 For further exploration of these narratives, see Zeiler (2005).

13 As seen, one interviewee did question this view but he framed it as a questioning by patients who had used PGD to women and men who had a high risk for a particular genetic disease, but who did not use PGD: 'I suspect they probably think that those couples have no right to have an affected child'. The reasoning of normality can also be further complicated, such as was done when some interviewees described PGD as a natural technology. If so, there were natural means to normal children and it was normal to want to use these natural technologies.

14 When interviewees' described the value of choice, they also often explicitly distanced themselves from the eugenics of the early twentieth century. At that time, interviewees commented, the heart of the matter was disease avoidance as such. Obligatory sterilisations were done in order to avoid the birth of children with certain diseases or with characteristics that was assumed to be non-desirable and possible to inherit. Women and (to a lesser extent) men were sterilised and they had no choice.

15 Koch and Nordahl-Svendsen (2005: 824) also argue that the knowledge created in genetic counselling situations and 'solutions' encompassed become the framework in which 'the problems' of being at risk for a genetic condition are created. Autonomous actors – patients – are created who consent 'to act responsibly with [disease] prevention as the almost inevitable result'.

16 It can also be noted that, according to the sociologist Tom Shakespeare (1998: 669), it is 'increasingly common' that clinicians use the term 'genetic disease' to refer to genetic conditions varying from cystic fibrosis to achondroplasia. The disability movement, Shakespeare says, contests this general labelling.

17 This number varies with different clinics.

18 One interviewee did hold that selection based on the knowledge of the genome of the particular embryo was ethically problematic and that it was a matter of going against Nature. Another interviewee did question pre-implantation genetic *screening* on the basis that it may become normal to search for embryos. For an exploration of this view, see Zeiler (2005).

19 I concur with those who hold that it is becoming more and more important to help couples discern and analyse their own experiences, values, assumptions and

ideas (see Dodds 2000); I also doubt that genetic counselling can ever be fully non-directive.

20 As an example of such a criticism, after having reviewed empirical data of interviews with kidney dialysis patients, first-person illness memoirs, studies of sociological ethnographies of bioethics as a practice within medicine as well as empirical studies of autonomy, Carl E. Schneider (1998) argued that many patients reject the burden of decision-making that is imposed on them. Instead, patients want more 'personal concern' and fewer decisions (to be distinguished from information) about treatment.

21 The exception is genetic diseases.

22 This makes the very notion of patient slightly misleading. Patients in everyday vocabulary often have a disease or an impairment that makes them contact a medical professional, though this is not always the case, as is clear in the whole field of delivery care. Furthermore, if pre-implantation genetic screening is used, neither of the partners need have a disease nor be a carrier of a disease, if infertility is not a consequence of a particular disease or is understood as a disease.

23 There is an important difference between the woman and man in the reproductive clinic, in terms of who will undergo most invasive treatment and be subject to most risks. Still, in homologous IVF, i.e. IVF without donor, both partners are physically involved in treatment, though the woman has the lion's share. In heterologous IVF, IVF with donor, both partners are also involved (but in another way) since both are needed to establish the need of a donor or donors.

24 Nikolas Rose (1999) discusses this view in a text in which he elaborates on Bourdieu's concept of governmentality.

References

Beachamp, T.L. and Childress, J.F. (2001) [1979] *Principles of Biomedical Ethics*, 5th edn, Oxford: Oxford University Press.

Bosch, X. (2004) 'UK criticized for embryo screening decision,' *Nature Medicine*, 10: 1266.

Bosk, C. (1993) 'The work-place ideology of genetic counselors,' in D.M. Bartel, B.S. LeRoy and A.L. Caplan (eds) *Prescribing Our Future: Ethical Challenges in Genetic Counselling*, New York: Alter De Gruyter.

Braude, P., Pickering, S., Flinter, F. and Ogilvie, C.M. (2002) 'Preimplantation genetic diagnosis,' *Nature Reviews Genetics*, 3: 941–53.

Corrigan, O. (2003) 'Empty ethics: the problem of informed consent,' *Sociology of Health and Illness*, 25: 768–92.

Cortazzi, M. (1993) *Narrative Analysis*, London: Falmer.

Denzin, N.K. (1989) *Interpretative Interactionism*, Newbury Park, CA: Sage Publications.

DHR (Swedish National Association for People with Mobility Impairments) (1998) *Remissyttrande över 'Genetik inom hälso- och sjukvården. En kunskapsöversikt och vägledning vid etiska bedömningar.'* Online. Available at: http://www.dhr.se/showFile.asp?objectld=2541 (accessed 1 March 2005).

DHR (Swedish National Association for People with Mobility Impairments) (2001) *Remissyttrande över Att spränga gränser – bioteknikens möjligheter och risker (SOU 2000:103). Slutbetänkandet av bioteknikkommittén. (Fördjupat yttrande).* Online. Available at: http://www.dhr.se/showFile.asp?objectld=2520 (accessed 1 March 2005).

Dodds, S. (2000) 'Choice and control in bioethics,' in C. Mackenzie and N. Stoljar (eds) *Relational Autonomy – Feminist Perspectives on Autonomy, Agency and the Social Self*, Oxford and New York: Oxford University Press.

Ettorre, E. (1999) 'Experts as "story-tellers" in reproductive genetics: exploring key issues,' *Sociology of Health and Illness*, 21: 539–59.

Faden, R. and Beauchamp, T. (1986) *A History and Theory of Informed Consent*, Oxford: Oxford University Press.

Franklin, S. (1997) *Embodied Progress: A Cultural Account of Assisted Conception*, London: Routledge.

Franklin, S. and Roberts, C. (forthcoming) *Born and Made: An Ethnography of Preimplantation Genetic Diagnosis*, Princeton, NJ: Princeton University Press.

Harris, J. (2000) 'Is there a coherent social conception of disability?,' *Journal of Medical Ethics*, 26: 95–100.

Harris, R. (1998) 'Genetic counselling and testing in Europe,' *Journal of the Royal College of Physicians of London*, 32: 335–8.

Herrenstein-Smith, B. (1981) 'Narrative versions, narrative theories,' in W. Mitchell (ed.) *On Narrative*, Chicago, IL: University of Chicago Press.

HFEA (Human Fertilisation and Embryology Authority) (2001) Report of the Pre-implantation Tissue Typing Policy Review. Online. Available at: http://www.hfea. gov.uk/AboutHFEA/HFEAPolicy/Pre-implantationtissuetyping (accessed 17 April 2005).

Hildt, E. (2002) 'Autonomy and freedom of choice in prenatal genetic diagnosis,' *Medicine, Health Care and Philosophy*, 5: 65–71.

Hoedemaekers, R. and ten Have, H. (1999) 'The concept of abnormality in medical genetics,' *Theoretical Medicine and Bioethics*, 20: 537–61.

Koch, L. and Nordahl-Svendsen, M. (2005) 'Providing solutions – defining problems: the imperative of disease prevention in genetic counselling,' *Social Science and Medicine*, 60: 823–32.

Labov, W. (1972) *Language in the Inner City: Studies in the Black Vernacular*, Philadelphia, PA: University of Pennsylvania Press.

Lebacqz, K. (1999) 'The ambiguities of "therapy" and their implications for the place of women and the disabled in a gene-focused society,' in A. Nordgren (ed.) *Gene Therapy and Ethics*, Uppsala: Uppsala University Press.

Legge 19 Febbraio 2004, n. 40, Norme in Materia di Procreazione Medicalmente Assistita [Italian Law on Assisted Reproductive Technologies, my translation from Italian]. Online. Available at: http://www.tecnobiosprocreazione.it/legge. php?menu=0 (accessed 29 April 2005).

Lippman, A. (1998) 'The politics of health: geneticization versus health promotion,' in S. Sherwin (ed.) *The Politics of Women's Health: Exploring Agency and Autonomy*, Philadelphia, PA: Temple University Press.

Lupton, D. (1997) 'Consumerism, reflexitivity, and the medical encounter,' *Social Science and Medicine*, 45: 373–81.

Marteau, T.M., Drake, H. and Bobrow, M. (1994a) 'Counselling following diagnosis of a fetal abnormality: the differing approaches of obstetricians, clinical geneticists, and genetic nurses,' *Journal of Medical Genetics*, 31: 864–7.

Marteau, T., Drake, H., Reid, M., Feijoo, M., Soares, M., Nippert, I., Nippert, P. and Bobrow, M. (1994b) 'Counselling following diagnosis of fetal abnormality: a comparison between German, Portuguese and UK geneticists,' *European Journal of Human Genetics*, 2: 96–102.

Meyers, D.T. (1989) *Self, Society, and Personal Choice*, New York: Columbia University Press.

Modell, J. (1989) 'Last chance babies: interpretations of parenthood in an in vitro fertilization program,' *Medical Anthropology Quarterly*, New Series, 3: 124–38.

Polyani, L. (1989) *Telling the American Story*, Cambridge, MA and London: MIT Press.

Raymond, J.G. (1995) *Women as Wombs: Reproductive Technologies and the Battle Over Women's Freedom*, North Melbourne: Spinifex Press.

Reindal, S.M. (2000) 'Disability, gene therapy and eugenics – a challenge to John Harris,' *Journal of Medical Ethics*, 26: 89–94.

Roberts, C. and Franklin, S. (2004) 'Experiencing new forms of genetic choice: findings from an ethnographic study of pre-implantation genetic diagnosis,' *Human Fertility*, 7: 285–93.

Rose, N. (1999) *The Powers of Freedom*, Cambridge: Cambridge University Press.

Rubio, C., Simón, C., Vidal, F., Rodrigo, L., Pehlivan, T., Remohí, J. and Pellicer, A. (2003) 'Chromosomal abnormalities and embryo development in recurrent miscarriage couples,' *Human Reproduction*, 18: 182–8.

Schneider, C.E. (1998) *The Practice of Autonomy: Patients, Doctors and Medical Decisions*, New York: Oxford University Press.

Shakespeare, T. (1998) 'Choices and rights: eugenics, genetics and disability equality,' *Disability and Society*, 13: 665–81.

Shakespeare, T. (1999) '"Losing the plot?" Medical and activist discourses of contemporary genetics and disability,' *Sociology of Health and Illness*, 21: 669–88.

Shakespeare, T. (2003) 'Rights, risks and responsibilities: new genetics and disabled people,' in S. Williams, L. Birke and G. Bendelow (eds) *Debating Biology: Sociological Reflections on Health, Medicine and Society*, London: Routledge.

SMER (Swedish National Council on Medical Ethics) (2004) Skrivelse om preimplantatorisk genetisk diagnostik. Online. Available at: http://www.smer.gov. se/index.htm?lang=sv&index=4&url=pgd.htm (accessed 30 April 2005).

SOU (1994/5) *18 Socialutskottets betänkande* (Swedish White Paper) Stockholm: Allmänna förlaget.

SOU (2004) *20 Genetik, etik, integritet* (Swedish White Paper on genetics, ethics and integrity) Stockholm: Allmänna förlaget.

The Lancet (2004) Editorial: 'Pre-implantation genetic diagnosis – for or against humanity?' *The Lancet*, 364:1729–30.

Thornhill, A.R., deDie-Smulders, C.E., Geraedts, J.P., Harper, J.C., Harton, G.L., Lavery, S.A., Moutou, C., Robinson, M.D., Schmutzler, A.G., Scriven P.N., Sermon, K.D. and Wilton, L. (2005) 'ESHRE PGD Consortium: best practice guidelines for clinical pre-implantation genetic diagnosis (PGD) and pre-implantation genetic screening (PGS),' *Human Reproduction*, 20: 35–48.

Wertz, D.C. and Fletcher, J.C. (1998) 'Eugenics is alive and well: a survey of genetic professionals around the world,' *Science in Context*, 11: 493–510.

Whyte, H. (1981) 'The value of narrativity in the representation of reality,' in W. Mitchell (ed.) *On Narrative*, Chicago, IL: University of Chicago Press.

Wolf, S. (1995) 'Beyond "genetic discrimination": toward the broader harm of geneticism,' *Journal of Law, Medicine and Ethics*, 23: 345–53.

Zeiler, K. (2005) 'Chosen Children and the Medical Profession. An empirical study and a philosophical analysis of moral aspects of pre-implantation genetic diagnosis and germ-line gene therapy,' Dissertation, Linköping Studies in Arts and Science 340, Linköping: Linköping University.

5 The normal baby-to-be

Lay and professional negotiations of the ultrasound image

Ann-Cristine Jonsson

Introduction

The image of the body is constantly shaped and re-shaped by the development of medical technology in late-modern society. Social scientists have increasingly paid attention to these changes in the image of the body, and have also argued that this leads to an uncertainty about what the body is (Shilling 1993; Williams 1997). Development within reproductive health, as well as within genetics, transplantation and plastic surgery, has created new possibilities for controlling the body, as well as to have it controlled by others. At the same time, this has encouraged an increased reflexivity about the body, and about how it can, or should, be reconstructed and controlled (Shilling 1993; Turner 1992). Ultrasound technology, as it is used within maternity health care, is one example of these new technologies, a technology that creates representations of the inner body and visualizes the expected baby.[1]

During the routine ultrasound scan, parts of the pregnant woman's body, and the expected baby, are visualized on a screen. This means that in the clinical situation, the health professionals as well as the parents-to-be[2] will encounter representations of the inner body and the expected baby. These representations do not speak for themselves, but have to be interpreted, explained and communicated in the clinical situation. The ultrasound technology thus confronts both parties with new problems related to the understanding of the body. Researchers have argued that the use of the routine ultrasound scan has introduced new conditions for how the individual can perceive the 'borders' of the body, and disrupted the traditional conception of inside and outside of the woman's body and of the pregnancy as 'an interior' experience (Petchesky 1987; Duden 1993). The visualization has resulted in a representation and a conception of the baby-to-be as separate and autonomous in relation to the woman, and the possibility to 'treat it as a patient already' (Petchesky 1987). Also, the medical assessment of the expected baby's health during pregnancy is no longer based primarily on the woman's experiences, but on the ultrasound technology (Georges 1996). The ultrasound technology has thus increased the possibility to control and survey the condition of the foetus, but it has also changed the general view of the relation between the baby-to-be and the pregnant woman, and given the woman an increasing responsibility for the health and wellbeing of the expected baby (Petchesky 1987; Lupton 1999).

The routine ultrasound scan, as other tests included in the programme designed for the surveillance of health during pregnancy, provides information that is supposed to increase the security during delivery and to detect deviancies in the woman's pregnancy and the expected baby's development at an early stage (Swedish National Board of Health and Welfare 1996).[3] Today, the routine ultrasound scan in Swedish maternity health care is carried out in gestational weeks 15–20.[4] The main purpose is to estimate gestational age, to detect multiple pregnancies and to localize the placenta, information that is used primarily to increase the security at delivery. The examination also offers opportunity to examine the foetus anatomy to detect malformations, something that has increasingly become a part of the routine ultrasound scan. Depending on more precisely when the scan is performed, the examination can also give additional information, for example about the sex of the expected baby. If the parents are aware that the examination can show the expected baby's sex, they also have to deal with the question of whether they want to ask for this information. The routine ultrasound scan is thus a surveillance-practice that has become more and more refined, as the capacity for early identifications of any deviancies in the normal development of the foetus continuously increases (Swedish Council on Technology Assessment in Health Care 1998).

At the same time as the ultrasound examination has resulted in a more refined medical control and surveillance of the pregnancy and the baby-to-be, it has also turned the experience of the expected baby into a more shared and public experience. The ultrasound scan is now regarded a milestone in parents' experiences of the pregnancy, and is also primarily looked upon as a social event (Sandelowski 1994; Draper 2002). To parents, the ultrasound image represents both a medical document and a photo of the baby (Sandelowski 1994). The ultrasound image is often treated as a first photo of the baby, and the ultrasound examination as a first encounter with the new family member (Sandelowski 1994; Mitchell and Georges 1997; Weir 1998).

The use of the routine ultrasound scan thus means that parents-to-be can see images, moving images, of the expected baby at an early stage of its development. Former generations of parents had only their own ideas, imaginations, and the baby's movements to rely on. The first contact with the expected baby was then established when the woman started to feel foetal movements, the 'quickening'. Today, the ultrasound examination seems to result in a 'technological quickening', which might change the 'order' through which parents establish a contact with the baby they are expecting (Petchesky 1987; Georges 1996; Mitchell and Georges 1997).

Different perspectives on the expected baby

The visualization of the expected baby during the routine ultrasound scan is likely to be perceived in different ways by the parents-to-be and the health care professionals respectively. It is the task of the professional, in this case the midwife, to interpret the medical meanings of the ultrasound image. Also, it is the professional who has the knowledge and skill to do this. The parents-to-be have to rely on the midwife's knowledge and skill to interpret the clinical meaning of the ultrasound image. At the same time they are anxious to have a confirmation that everything is fine with the baby (Green 1994).

In theoretical terms it is possible to say that the encounter between the midwife and the parents is an encounter between two different *perspectives*, the midwife's professional perspective and the parents' everyday perspective. Here, perspective refers to having a certain attitude or a certain approach to the situation or 'what is going on', and is thus related to the concept 'voice', as defined by Mishler (1984). The professional perspective is characterized by a distinctive goal-orientation, related to the fact that the midwife has certain tasks to perform. It is not primarily curiosity or fascination in the presence of the unborn baby that is important to her, but the critical examination of what she can see on the screen. The midwife will have to compare what she sees on the screen with clinical standards, in order to discover any deviance. Thus, the midwife's attitude to the interaction with the parents is oriented towards the clinical task and the critical investigation of the image of the expected baby on the ultrasound screen.

The everyday perspective is distinguished by a different attitude. Here, the expected baby is typically placed within a biographical context. The baby is first of all a part of the parents individual and joint life-projects, as a couple and as parents-to-be, not a question as to whether it corresponds with certain clinical standards or not. Here, the parent perspective refers to how the expected baby is placed within a biographical context. This means that what is seen on the monitor from a parent perspective first of all is interpreted in a non-critical way. As a consequence, any worry that the expected baby is not 'normal' will be understood primarily in an everyday and not a medical sense. The parents' interaction with each other and the midwife is in this sense likely to be characterized by a non-directedness, that is the parents' attitude to the interaction is not directed by any pre-set medical task. The parents will first of all see an image of the future baby, and not an image of a foetus to be assessed according to medical norms.

The ultrasound examination can in this sense be described as an encounter between two different perspectives, the midwife's professional perspective and the parents' everyday perspective. The purpose of this chapter is to explore how the issue of the expected baby's normality is communicated and negotiated between these different perspectives during the routine ultrasound examination.

The negotiation and construction of normality through the ultrasound examination

To shed light on the communication and negotiation of normality, I will draw on an analysis of twelve observed and audio-taped ultrasound examinations which are part of a larger empirical study of how the ultrasound image is communicated and ascribed meaning in the interaction between the midwife and the parents-to-be (Jonsson 2004). The participants in these twelve examinations were couples, expecting their first or second child together. (Some of them had children in earlier relationships.) They all came for routine ultrasound scans, and none of them had any illnesses or complications related to the pregnancy that was known about beforehand.

One characteristic feature of the clinical encounter is that it is structured by distinct phases that recur in every meeting (Drew and Heritage 1992). As the structure, and the phases of the encounter, is shaped by the tasks that the professional has to carry out, these phases will vary between different types of clinical settings (Baggens 2002; Hydén and Mishler 1999; Silverman 1987; Mishler 1984). The routine ultrasound examination proved, similar to other clinical encounters, to be clearly structured by the professional tasks of the midwife (Jonsson 2004). I have earlier described how the typical ultrasound examination can be seen as structured into four distinct phases (ibid.). The first phase, the 'initial control', is a critical part of the examination during which the midwife finds out if the baby is healthy or not. The midwife uses the image on the screen first of all as a tool to perform her professional tasks. During the second phase, 'measurements', the midwife also uses the screen image primarily as a diagnostic tool, but she also starts to interpret the image to the parents. Proceeding to the next phase, 'showing the baby's body parts', the midwife tries to make what is shown on the screen understandable to the parents. During the last phase, 'taking the baby's picture', the midwife tries to capture a picture that depicts the unborn baby in a 'baby-like' position that resembles a portrait when she prints a paper copy of the screen image.[5]

Here, I will follow these phases of the ultrasound examination, phase by phase, to explore the ways in which normality is negotiated and established in the interaction between the midwife's professional perspective and the parent's everyday perspective, through the ultrasound examination. First, I will explore how the issue of normality is typically managed between the different perspectives of the midwife and the parents in the clinical encounter, and then look at how a suspicion about a potential deviance in the baby's health is dealt with.

Localization and confirmation of the baby's existence

In the first phase of the ultrasound examination, 'initial control', the fact that the baby exists is confirmed by the midwife. In Example 1, we will follow Lena and Lennart and their midwife through this phase. These parents-to-be are expecting their first baby, and this is their first ultrasound examination together (Lena had a scan in the ninth gestational week, when Lennart was not present). Here, we have all just entered the examination room and the midwife has shown the parents where to take a seat, Lena on the bunk and Lennart on a chair which is placed next to the bunk. From these seats, they face the screen for the parents to look at. The midwife takes her seat behind her own screen, which cannot be seen by the parents. The midwife then starts the ultrasound examination.

Example 1

MIDWIFE: There now, now this will feel a little cold and sticky and you'll see
— do you think that it [the screen] is correctly angled towards you? can
you see it when you sit like that or?

LENA: Ooh yes

MIDWIFE: Yes because you will have to look at that one yourselves, but I
have the same picture on this slightly smaller screen in front of me then
(LENA: hum) now what I'll do first I'll look through and check and see
what I see and then I'll explain to you, you probably understand quite
well but, I will explain to you when I have finished looking (...) I'll be
rather quiet to begin with.

(the midwife scans for eight seconds)

LENA: Do you understand [to Lennart] can you see what it is? [laughter] ooh
[quietly] [the midwife scans for 23 seconds]

LENA: One can see the heart anyway [quietly].

What we see here is that the midwife sets the terms for the encounter, by deciding who will sit where and what shall be done, terms that are related to her professional tasks. She starts the examination proper and then conducts a first preliminary check of the unborn baby. In this first phase of the examination, it is the midwife who has the initiative. She structures the interaction by placing the man on a chair, and the woman on the bunk in front of their screen, and herself behind 'her' screen. But the midwife also structures the interaction by telling the parents what she will do during the examination. She does this by using a verbal phrase that is also used in the other examinations as well: 'now, what I will do is that I will first have a look and check and see what I see, and then I will explain to you'.

The midwife here governs the interaction in several ways. She divides her own and the parents looking at separate screens through pointing out to the parents, verbally as well as with gestures, that they should direct their attention towards their own screen and that she will look at her screen. She also tells the parents that she will initially be busy carrying out her first check-ups and therefore stay silent, and that she will not start to tell the parents about her interpretation of the image on the screen until later. Also, she governs the interaction by being silent. In addition, a consequence of how the midwife and the parents are placed in the room is that it is impossible for them to watch each other's facial expressions when looking on the screen placed in front of them.

After this, the midwife starts to perform the ultrasound examination with her attention directed towards the information she gets from the image on the screen. Lena and Lennart stay silent to begin with and look at the images of the expected baby that appear on their screen, which may be seen as accepting the form of interaction that the midwife has initiated. After a while Lena asks Lennart in a quiet voice if he can see what it is that is being shown on the screen, but he continues to stay silent and does not answer. They look at the screen in silence for a moment, while the midwife continues to carry out her tasks. Lena then states that 'one can see the heart anyway'. So, at the same time as the midwife is carrying out her tasks, the parents are busy looking at the screen.

When the midwife carries out this first assessment the parents typically remain silent. However, in some cases the parents start to talk between themselves about what they see on the screen, while the midwife carries out the first check-up. This happens for example during the ultrasound examination of Monika and Morgan. Morgan has two children previously, and now they are expecting their first baby together. Before this examination, Monika has had one ultrasound scan as part of medical examination in the eighth gestational week.

Example 2

MIDWIFE: Then I'll do like this now first I'll look myself and measure and do what I am supposed to do (MONIKA: yeah) and then I'll show you some more later
MONIKA: Uhm
MORGAN: Absolutely
MONIKA: This is fun [quietly]
MORGAN: Yeah I think so too actually [quietly]
    [the midwife scans for six seconds]
MONIKA: Oh dear, look, a leg, what fun [quietly]
MORGAN: What did you say? [quietly]
MONIKA: Oh dear this is a leg, I think, and then an arm to the left now it disappeared
MORGAN: So it's moving [laughter] it's moving the whole time
MONIKA: Apparently
MIDWIFE: Uhum you can't catch up
MORGAN: There, there, there was a head there, huh?
MIDWIFE: [laughter].

Here, the parents talk to each other quietly, and they do not turn to the midwife but to each other for a confirmation of their interpretation of the image on the screen. By communicating with each other in this way, directed away from the midwife and quietly, the parents re-structure the participant relations that the midwife has initially established. Monika and Morgan turn to each other, as a couple, but do not turn to the midwife. As a result, the midwife for a moment becomes a spectator and an audience to the parents' dialogue with each other, and the everyday interpretation of the images on the screen dominates the interaction.

Characteristic of the midwife's way of managing the image on the screen in this phase is thus that she neither comments on the image herself, nor shares her clinical interpretation of the image with the parents; she stays silent. In addition to this way of establishing an order for the interaction that lets her carry out her tasks in an efficient way, this also works as a way to handle the issue of the baby's normality. During this phase, the midwife carries out a first preliminary assessment of the normality of the pregnancy and the foetus, which is to check if the foetus is properly situated in the uterus, the number of foetuses and if the expected baby is alive. Until this is done, the normality of the pregnancy and the expected baby is still to be assessed. During this part of the examination, the ultrasound image is not commented upon until the baby's existence is localized and confirmed. At the same time, the parents look attentively at the screen and try to understand what they see from their parental perspective. It also happens, as we see in the case of Monika and Morgan, that the parents comment on the parts of the baby that they can perceive, which can also be understood as a way to reflect on the baby, that it is there and possible to see, and that the baby has legs, arms, feet, etc., that is, what normal babies should have.

Measuring the baby

The next phase of the examination is constituted by the midwife's measurements of the expected baby. She continues to carry out the check-ups and the measurements that are included in the examination, which also includes an estimate of the date of delivery. In the following example the midwife initiates this phase of the examination by telling the parents that she will now begin to measure the expected baby's leg, something that is related to the calculation of the date of delivery.

Example 3

MIDWIFE: Oops (…) so, then I'll measure a leg then we see the thigh rather clearly here (LENA: mm) (…) when approximately do you expect the delivery to take place? Is it in July or?

LENA: Yes, the twenty-third

MIDWIFE: Uhum

[the midwife scans for ten seconds]

MIDWIFE: It was estimated from your period then or?

LENA: Yes (MIDWIFE: yes) or yes, of course you did (an ultrasound)

MIDWIFE: Yeah, that's right, okay, exactly. We did the estimation a bit from that maybe (LENA: yeah) (...) this is the head seen from above (LENA: uhum) this is between the fingers [inaudible] (LENA: uhum)
[the midwife scans for 19 seconds]

MIDWIFE: Do you see the face (LENA: yes) [inaudible] eye, eye, it is almost laughing (LENA: yes) [laughter] the mouth (...)

LENA: Oh dear, oh no, that's cool

MIDWIFE: [laughter].

At the same time as the midwife performs the measurement, she starts to interpret the image on the screen to the parents. The midwife shifts between these tasks by first telling the parents about the check-up she is going to carry out, and then what they see on the screen: 'so, then I will measure a leg', and 'so we see the thigh rather clearly'. So, unlike in the first phase of the examination, the midwife now comments on what they see on the screen. This also means that the midwife directs the parents' looking at the screen with her talk and with the aid of the computer-arrow.

Example 4

MIDWIFE: Now I'll measure this one crosswise

MORGAN: It's, it's the head you've got there?

MIDWIFE: It's the head I'm measuring, right

MONIKA: I would have said it was the tummy! [quietly] [giggles]

MORGAN: What did you say?

MONIKA: I would have said it is the tummy [giggles]

MORGAN: [laughter].

When the midwife performs these measurements she 'freezes' the image on the screen. This means that when she measures the baby's head, it is seen as a still image. Her way of measuring, from temple to temple, results in an image of the head in cross-section, from above. The image on the screen then resembles an anatomical picture of the brain. The midwife repeatedly comments on this still image. She explains that the non-moving image on the screen does not signify anything abnormal. The way the midwife tries to make the image understandable can also be understood as a way to avoid worries about something being wrong with the baby that could be triggered by what the parents see on the screen.

Also, the midwife always asks the woman about the calculated date of delivery according to previous dating, as we see in Example 3. In most cases, a dating has already been done earlier in the pregnancy, which means that the midwife, as well as the parents, already has a date to relate to. The midwife, in her conversation with the parents, always comments on the estimated date of delivery that she arrives at in relation to any former date.

In those cases when this new date corresponds with earlier estimations, the midwife does not say much about this. But when the midwife arrives at a new date she always tries to explain this to the parents. In these cases, the new date means that the parents have to move the previously estimated date of delivery forwards or backwards in time. The estimation of the date of delivery is here an issue that takes up a lot of time in the conversation, and is dealt with at length. For example, the midwife can explain that the discrepancy between a former date and the date that she has estimated might be due to the inaccuracy of the estimation method. A changed date of delivery can also be used to 'explain' the woman's present health and well-being.

Example 5

NILS: Oh dear (...) now you measure the head huh?

MIDWIFE: Now I measure the head yes – from side to side, we shall now (...) it turns out to be the sixteenth of August, what did you say?

NINA: The tenth!

MIDWIFE: The tenth. Okay so a couple of days later then, this might explain all this feeling of sickness and this miserable state of things and that you have had it for such a long time, that you actually haven't been that (...) though we perhaps (...) did we say the sixteenth from the beginning as well?

NINA: No we said the tenth

MIDWIFE: Okay so then it is a little later then (NINA: okay) there now we shall see.

In all conversations these kinds of changes between earlier and new dates are treated with caution and explained as something normal. So, also in this phase of the examination the image on the screen first of all works as a diagnostic tool for the midwife and the interpretations of the ultrasound image are made from her professional perspective.

Visualizing the normal baby

After having done the first measurment of the expected baby, the midwife changes her approach to the image on the screen. She now starts to interpret and explain the image to the parents. This shift in how the image is handled in the interaction is also possible to discern in the midwife's talk.

Example 6

MIDWIFE: But then I shall point to you here then (...) let's see if you can get that down just a little little more here (LENA: yes) [inaudible] (LENA: yes) then it is like this, we see I shall just put a cross here, can you see that it is a cross here?

LENA: Uhum (…)

MIDWIFE: Your bladder isn't very full, you don't need to go to the toilet [laughter]

LENA: No, not much

MIDWIFE: [laughter] But it should be here somewhere but one can't see it very well, this is the uterus then, and in the front one can see the placenta, that's the slightly thicker wall that (LENA: yes) is placed like this. Oh dear what a speed it has, can you see the legs moving down here? (LENA: yes) [laughter] yes it is the knees here (LENA: yes) and then you can see that the feet far out in that direction are kicking, it is kicking a lot now

LENA: Mm maybe they can feel that

MIDWIFE: Do you?

LENA: No but he or she

MIDWIFE: Right [laughter] it might.

During this part of the examination the midwife also changes her way of using the computer-arrow on the screen. She now starts to apply it as a pointer, instead of as a measuring apparatus. As the midwife has the command of the computer-arrow, she can to some extent decide what the parents should look at and what images should be commented on. In this sense, the use of the computer-arrow also works as a way to guide the parents' vision. However, the midwife obviously cannot avoid that the parents might choose to comment on something completely different from what she tries to point out, and maybe in that way change the perspective on what is being seen on the screen.

The midwife's comments are largely focused on the image on the screen. Her interpretations of the image are primarily explanations of what the image shows, something that becomes evident in the way she phrases her comments. She frequently uses expressions such as 'this is', 'here one can see' and 'then you can see', as is demonstrated in the following example.

Example 7

MIDWIFE: Yes, exactly look at the cross here now so we can have a little look at the baby [quietly] so this is the chin here and then up towards the mouth and nose. There's a nice profile here (MARIA: [giggles]) and then the forehead, back towards the neck, here the back is in this direction, the bottom upwards and then we have the legs here, though we can't see them properly right now (MARIA: right) and then this is the stomach, right then I'll turn this one on again so that it becomes mobile again [the image has been 'frozen'] right, then here we see that the heart beats.

The midwife points out parts of the baby, such as the face, nose, chin, profile, neck, back, bottom and legs. But besides showing what can actually be seen on the screen, the midwife also alerts the parents to various body *functions*, such as when she points out that it is possible to see the heart beat. In this way, the interpretation of the image also shows the functions of the baby's inner organs and that the baby is alive. This is something we also can see in the next example.

Example 8

MIDWIFE: Here you can see the heart clearly (OLIVIA and OSKAR: yeah) can you see (OLIVIA and OSKAR: yes) the heart chambers too, it's like a little cross, there is one line here and one line there (OLIVIA: yes) can you see that there's a black spot there (OLIVIA: yes) that's the stomach and that's the heart [inaudible] (OLIVIA and OSKAR: uhum)
[the midwife continues to show other body parts].

In addition to commenting on the image with reference to body functions, the midwife here also comments on the *structure of the body*, when she shows the structure of the heart by pointing out the heart chambers: 'it's like a little cross'. Another typical pattern is the pointing out of the *completeness* of the baby's body.

Example 9

MIDWIFE: And here one can see the bottom and here one can see the bladder here one can see the thigh and the thigh and the knee and the knee, now I'm twisting this thing and then one can see the lower leg, here is one lower leg there is the other lower leg and then there is the foot far out there (OLIVIA: uhum) it might perhaps be a little difficult to see when you're not used to looking at these small details so that's why you almost have to do like this (OLIVIA: yes) one can see it from a little distance (OSKAR: yes) there you have the feet or the legs, to the left and the head to the right then
OLIVIA: Yes, exactly
OSKAR: Uhum.

Whenever an arm, hand, leg, knee or foot is shown, the midwife looks for an image that makes it possible for the parents to see the complementary body part as well. Also, in those cases where the other arm, leg or foot cannot be seen, the midwife explicitly comments that it does exist. Other body parts that are pointed out are the expected baby's thighs, hips, arms, hands and fingers. When the hands or feet are shown, the question of numbers, numbers of fingers, hands, etc., will in most cases be a topic of interest.

Example 10

MIDWIFE: A foot, can you see the whole foot sole here, and then this is the
heel and then the toes are here (LENA: yeah)

LENA: It's got five toes? [laughter]

MIDWIFE: Yes we shall see they are rather small so that, smaller than three
millimetres almost (LENA: yes)

MIDWIFE: [inaudible]

[the midwife scans for ten seconds]

LENA: I don't know if I'm making this up but I think I can feel it

MIDWIFE: I'm sure you do, I'm sure you could have felt, but you never know
what it is for sure (LENA: no) later on you will understand, but the first
time it could be a bubbly tummy or anything, I'm sure you have felt it
that's what I think (…) it's not very far away to you (…) you don't have
very much in between

[the midwife shows the distance between the baby's feet and the inner
surface of the womb].

In this example, we also see that the interpretations of the image alert
the parents to questions concerning the baby's health and normality. Lena's
statement might be understood as a question about the number of toes and
thus as a worry. She does not ask straightforwardly if the foot looks normal
and if all the fingers are there, but chooses a weaker form, which is typical of
how parents phrase their concerns. The midwife always assures the parents
that all the body parts are there, and explains that they also will be able to
see these body parts. In most cases she uses the zoom-function to try to find
an image that will make all the toes or fingers visible. In this way the midwife
tries to help the parents to 'see' the image on the screen. She is also showing
that the expected baby is 'complete' and normal, and she makes a special
point of showing that every body part is there. In Example 10, when the
expected baby's feet are shown, the midwife makes an effort to bring her
own professional perspective on the image of the expected baby in line with
the woman's everyday understanding and questions about the baby. She does
this for example by carefully and with precision helping the woman to 'see'
the baby's toes.

The midwife also explains how the inner organs might be recognized on
the screen. In the next example, she speaks about 'black spots', and then tells
the parents what organ or body part can be identified on the screen, in this
case the stomach.

Example 11

MIDWIFE: Then it is the head that we have got it is this [inaudible] that was
what we saw then and the heart, quite right too that you saw the chest
in here in (…) (LENA: uhum) there, those black spots under there, is the

stomach (LENA: uhum) and down there one can see the bladder of the foetus then (...) its bladder is almost more full then yours!

LENA: Yes [laughter].

In explaining how the inner organs can be recognized, the midwife switches between professional and everyday expressions. From her professional perspective the black nuance is not only a black spot that can be recognized as an inner organ, but also an indication of the fact that the inner organs work as they should. The stomach would not be possible to discern as a black unless the baby was able to swallow and digest foetal water.

Beside these interpretations of the image on the screen, the midwife also points out the expected baby's *movements*, and from what angle the parents see these movements. When she speaks about the expected baby's movements the midwife not only demonstrates that the baby moves, but she also speaks about the movements in terms of speed and energy (also see Example 6 above). Here, the midwife's interpretation of the image on the screen changes. She goes from interpreting the image in a professional way, mainly focusing on confirming that the different parts of the expected baby seen on the screen are in accordance with the medical norms for foetal development, to a more everyday interpretation of the image, referring to the social and psychological characteristics of the expected baby. This can be seen also in Example 11, where the midwife jokes about the baby's overfilled bladder.

In other words, the midwife shifts perspective and presents the image on the screen from what could be called a parental perspective, to make it possible for the parents to identify the visual patterns as their baby. In doing this, the midwife starts out from her professional capacity to see and ascribe meaning and content to the different elements of the image to help the parents to see. What she first sees is the anatomical structure of the baby's body, and that is what she focuses on. At the same time she shifts to commenting on the image from an everyday perspective. This shift is demonstrated for instance in Examples 6 and 11, where the midwife, by laughing, indicates that what she says should be interpreted in a particular way; that she is joining the mother in 'seeing' the unborn baby from an everyday perspective.

As we have seen in the examples the interpretation of the ultrasound image is not an unproblematic task, especially as the question of deviance is always there as a potential threat. The ultrasound image of the baby is shown and interpreted by the midwife mainly with a focus on making it comprehensible to the parents. This 'showing of the baby' both in a professional as well as an everyday perspective, might also be understood as a way of visualizing a *normal* baby. This is accomplished by the pointing out of body parts, from top to toe, identifying all the vital inner organs and their proper functioning and structure, and that the baby's anatomy is fine. By 'translating' the image in this way, the midwife implicitly confirms to the parents, without verbally telling them, that from a professional point of view there are no signs of any abnormality.

Pictorial evidence of the normal baby

In the last phase of the examination, 'taking the baby's picture', the midwife usually starts by asking the parents whether they have any questions and if they have seen what they expected to see. The midwife also gives the parents an opportunity to ask additional questions about the image. This also seems to function as a way to indicate to the parents that the examination is coming to an end.

Example 12

MIDWIFE: Do you have any questions now? Now when you have seen this?
LENA: No
MIDWIFE: Does it look the way you thought it would, or?
LENA: Yes
LENNART: Just about
MIDWIFE: Just about (...) okay
LENNART: How big is it now?
MIDWIFE: Well, if one measures [the midwife continues to explain how she estimates the baby's length].

Here, the woman, Lena, answers the midwife's question by saying that her questions have been answered and that the visualization of the baby-to-be looks something like she had expected. The man, Lennart, states that he has by and large seen what he expected. He then asks how big the baby is at the moment. The midwife explains how the size might be calculated, and then tells them the results of her measurements, the estimated date of delivery. The midwife then prints a couple of paper copies of the ultrasound image.

Example 13

[prints out paper copies from the ultrasound apparatus]
MIDWIFE: Yes it looks fine (...) as one [inaudible]
LENA: Okay (...)
MIDWIFE: Can you see the profile?
LENA: Yes
MIDWIFE: It's moving its mouth a little [quietly]
LENA: Yes
[the midwife scans for 7 seconds]
MIDWIFE: The fingers there and the nose here, the hand by the mouth [inaudible]

[the midwife prints out another paper copy]

MIDWIFE: Here you can see four fingers and a thumb here [quietly] (LENA: yes) you can see that (LENA: yes) it is almost as if you could believe that this is the mouth [quietly] (LENA: uhum)

[the midwife scans for 10 seconds]

MIDWIFE: Uhum well then, then I am done (LENA: yes) I will mail you a report later on.

The midwife declares that 'yes it looks good'. Statements like 'it looks good', 'everything looks fine so far' or 'it looks fine', are also found in the other cases during this last phase of the examination. These utterances can have various meanings referring to the image as such, as well as to the result of the whole examination. As no further references are made to the image on the screen in this example, it is likely that the utterance refers to the result from the foetal-diagnostic part of the examination, and implicitly confirms that everything looks normal. It is less likely that the utterance refers to the estimated date of delivery, as this is always discussed separately.

It is thus possible to understand these forms of utterance from the midwife as a summing-up of the examination from a professional perspective: medically she has not discovered any problems or deviancies to communicate to the parents, normality is confirmed. Sometimes, more explicit references are made to normality.

Example 14

MIDWIFE: It looks completely normal as far as I can judge it here (KATRIN: uhum) I don't see anything that deviates anywhere but it is a normal foetus (KATRIN: yes) and the size as I said is also okay, then as I said on the whole (KATRIN: yes) uhum it's lying down there wiggling its head

KATRIN: Yes, it is so small [quietly]

MIDWIFE: Yes!

MIDWIFE: Now then, do you have any questions now?

KATRIN: No.

Here, the midwife concludes that the image of the expected baby looks normal. The typical pattern is however that the midwife does not specify what it is that looks fine or normal when she tells the parents about the results of the examination. Interestingly, in this example the midwife fairly soon leaves her professional perspective again and moves over to show, not the foetus, but a picture of the baby with a profile, fingers and mouth etc.

Another typical pattern in this example is that the midwife tries to create an image that is 'worth seeing', something that resembles a portrait, for instance by pointing out the profile. The image is thus translated into an everyday perspective. Finally, the midwife closes the whole examination by again shifting to a professional approach when she informs the parents-to-be about the next examination at the ante-natal clinic.

In this fashion normality is finally established and communicated in this last phase of the examination. The midwife tells the parents about her results of the measurements, by presenting the estimated date of delivery, sometimes combined with comments about the image on the screen, such as 'it looks fine' (albeit sometimes without any explicit reference to normality at all). Here, the clinical evaluation of the baby-to-be and the pregnancy is again accompanied by a biographical contextualization of the ultrasound image of the baby, as the midwife translates the image to an everyday perspective and hands over a paper copy, a photo, of the expected baby to the parents. In this last phase of the examination, as well as in the previous one, a change occurs as the image is increasingly being interpreted within a biographical context.

Management of potential deviance

Sometimes, an unexpected outcome can create a potential problem during the ultrasound examination. In these situations, the parties have to manage this potential problem in the interaction. Parents-to-be probably always feel some kind of worry that something might be wrong with the baby they are expecting. These worries can be latent in the interaction during the whole ultrasound scan. In the ultrasound examinations that I observed in this study, no serious deviancies were identified. In one case, however, the midwife did get a measurement that did not fit with what was expected. This turned out to have completely different consequences for the two parties. To the midwife it meant that she has to check this measurement once again, even if it did not have any serious clinical consequences. To the parents, on the other hand, their worries were aroused when the midwife first told them about the result as a not-normal measurement.

Renate and Rikard, who are expecting their second baby, are having their first ultrasound scan in this pregnancy. In the same way as in the other cases, the midwife in the initial phrase speaks about how she will arrange the examination. During the measurement phase, she continues to conduct her check-up at the same time as she asks the parents about the former estimated date of delivery. She continues with her tasks and talks about how she now measures the baby's thighs, and points out both legs.

Example 15

MIDWIFE: It's the thigh that I want to get hold of, now then (...) there you can see both legs how they reach out like this
RIKARD: From the back then, or from the side?
MIDWIFE: Not quite, right now you can see, then in that corner from the side
[the midwife scans for nine seconds]

MIDWIFE: Two [quietly] then I have to check the checklist, because I didn't
get the measurement quite right [clears her throat]
[the midwife turns around and picks up the checklist and looks at it]
MIDWIFE: Now let's see
[the midwife then gets up from her chair and walks towards a bench
next to her and opens a folder].

In contrast to the other cases, where the midwife typically performs the
measurement and talks about what she checks without any further comments
on the measurements, the midwife here tells the parents that she has to check
this measurement again, because it does not correspond to the expected
outcome. 'I didn't get the measurement quite right', she says. Similar to
what happens in the other examinations the midwife does not talk about
what she is doing in any detail. In this sense she downplays the information
she gives to the parents.

Example 16

RIKARD: What did you say, did you get one?
MIDWIFE: See twenty-nine twenty-three
[browses through a folder with measurements standing next to the bench
where the researcher sits]
MIDWIFE: Twenty-three sixteen, thanks
[the researcher takes the folder as the midwife tries to put it back on the
bench]
RIKARD: Twenty-three what's that?
MIDWIFE: Well that is the head measurement
RIKARD: What did you say? [inaudible]
MIDWIFE: Yes just wait two seconds [laughter]
RIKARD: Yes of course
MIDWIFE: Fourteen plus three yes I understand that you are eager, I will just
check, I got a measurement that I'm not satisfied with so I have to go to
the hand-top
[sits with the hand-top in the hand]
MIDWIFE: Plus three [quietly] and then we say the twenty-third of September
and yes then it differs two days there you had got the twenty-fifth there
so it corresponds very well then
RIKARD: It does, does it?
MIDWIFE: Perfect to the time of pregnancy yes yes (…) it does so.

Rikard immediately asks what the midwife said and obviously wants to
know more: 'what did you say, did you get one?' The midwife then starts
to calculate, aided by her checklist, and in this way avoids answering his
questions. Rikard repeats one of the last figures that the midwife has spelled

out, and asks what is meant by that figure, 'twenty-three what's that?', and once again asks, 'what did you say?'

What happens here is that the midwife asks Rikard to wait and excuses herself by telling him once more that she has got a measurement that she is not satisfied with. The midwife then tries to avoid the question of the potentially deviant result of her measurement in various ways. Just as in the initial phase of the examination, the midwife does not share her clinical interpretation of the image with the parents. When the midwife presents the date of delivery that she has arrived at, she emphasizes the correspondence with her measurements, and she points out that this new date corresponds very well with earlier calculations: 'then it differs two days there you had got the twenty-fifth there so it corresponds very well then'. The midwife goes on to argue that it corresponds very well: 'perfect to the time yes yes it does'. Immediately afterwards she continues to explain to the parents which parts of the baby's body can be seen on the screen, which can also be understood as a way of leaving the topic of potentially deviant results. In these ways, she downplays the threat against the expected baby's normality, and neutralizes the deviant measurement. In this case, normality is not an issue that the midwife discusses with the parents when it is questioned and dubious.

Discussion and concluding comments

So, how is the expected baby's normality communicated and negotiated as part of the examination of the ultrasound image? As the analysis of these ultrasound examinations indicates, normality is an issue that the parties deal with throughout the examination. One could say that through the different ways the ultrasound image is interpreted, a confirmation of normality is achieved. During the first phase of the examination, the pregnancy and the expected baby's existence is still to be confirmed. This is reflected also in the way the midwife leaves the ultrasound image un-commented until the baby is localized and she has confirmed that the baby exists. While this is going on, the midwife does not discuss her professional tasks, or her clinical interpretation of the ultrasound image, in any explicit way. At the same time, the parents-to-be watch the screen attentively and try to understand what they see from their perspective. The comments that the parents make can be understood as reflections on the fact that the baby is actually there and can be seen. This confirmation of the fact that the baby exists can be seen as a first step in a confirmation of a normal pregnancy.

Another way of managing the issue of normality occurs in the following phase of the examination, where the midwife begins to explain what she is measuring to the parents. Here, she starts to talk about, and explain to the parents what she is measuring, and also what part of the baby they see on the screen. The measurements are continuously commented on as related to the norms for a normal pregnancy and the development of a healthy and normal baby. Also, the estimated date of delivery, which is the outcome of her measurements, is commented on as expected or according to the norms. Even differences between calculated dates of delivery are commented on as being within normal variation.

An additional way of managing normality can be seen in the next phase of the examination, when the midwife tries to make the image comprehensible for the parents, by showing the baby's body parts as well as the structure and function of vital organs. The midwife here changes from a professional perspective, where the purpose is to confirm that the expected baby follows the medical norms, to an everyday perspective as she interprets the image with references to the characteristics of the baby. As she interprets the ultrasound image from a professional as well as an everyday perspective, the midwife visualizes a normal and healthy baby and also confirms normality rhetorically.

This way of combining the two perspectives on the image can been seen again towards the end of the examination. Here, the midwife first presents the estimated date of delivery. She also communicates her summing-up of the examination from a professional perspective by stating that everything looks fine, sometimes without any explicit reference to normality. She then changes her way of interpreting of the image, and comments on the image as related to the biographical context of the family. Finally, she hands over a paper copy of the ultrasound image, a photo that shows the expected baby. Together, these ways of handling the image provide pictorial evidence of the normal child.

The issue of normality is thus not explicitly talked about from within a professional perspective. *What*, more precisely, the midwife is examining, is rarely talked about during the examination. Instead, normality is *visualized* as she interprets the image to the parents. The typical pattern is that the midwife shows the parents the baby with all body parts and everything that functions as it should – but this is not talked about as a check-up of normality. Normality is simply shown. This might be understood as a way to avoid worrying parents-to-be. Instead of talking and explaining the different assessments of the baby, the baby is shown, and the parents are left to raise questions if they want to. This way of managing the assessment of the expected baby's normality has many similarities with the 'indirect' strategies that have been demonstrated in earlier studies of how professionals manage health surveillance practices in situations where the examination in itself might evoke (groundless) worry (Olin Lauritzen and Sachs 2001; Bredmar and Linell 1999; Adelswärd and Sachs 1996; Strong 1979).

A similar way of handling normality is used when a potential deviance is found. In this study, no serious deviancies from normality were identified. However, it did happen that the midwife got a measurement that did not fit with the norm. When confronted with this type of deviant measurement, the midwife does not comment on her assessment until she has completed all the measurements she needs to come to a conclusion. When presenting the results, the midwife typically emphasizes the measurements do correspond with what is expected, and quickly moves on to show the baby on the screen. This might also be interpreted as two ways to neutralize the initially deviant measurement. The general pattern also when confronted with a potential deviance is that this assessment is carried out within the professional perspective, and that the issue of normality is not raised for discussion by the midwife.

In this study, the ultrasound examination has been analysed as an encounter between a professional and an everyday perspective. The way the midwife constantly moves between her own professional and the parents' everyday perspective is striking. Of particular interest is the way she comments on the image on the screen and the way she is 'taking the perspective of the other'. By translating her professional interpretation of the ultrasound image into the parents' everyday perspective she helps the parents to organize how and what they see. At the same time, by taking the perspective of the parents, the midwife can see something else in the image than for instance the anatomical structure of the baby that belongs to the professional perspective. One could say that the parents help the midwife to see the image of a baby that within a fairly short period of time will become a member of a family, a family that in the ultrasound examination literally tries to catch a sight of its new member. The meaning of the image is not given – not least because of the qualities of the image on the screen – but has to be actively created by, among other things, organizing and interpreting the image. Through this process, the interpretation and understanding of the image that appears on the screen is negotiated.

These negotiations and interpretations of the image of the expected baby also point to an interesting condition for our vision, opened up by the health technology. Due to her professional capacity to interpret the image, the midwife directs the attention of the parents towards the aspects of the image that are being explained during the ultrasound examination. The parents are in this sense, as Duden (1993) has argued, 'shown' what they should see in the medical image, by the midwife, the expert. The midwife chooses what should be shown, and what should be explained, for example to show a normally developed heart with a clearly discernible four-chamber picture or a waving hand. In the clinical situation there is consequently a tension between the ultrasound image as a diagnostic tool and the ultrasound image as an image of the expected baby.

What is also indicated is that through the ultrasound image that the parents are confronted with in the clinical context, they are in various ways forced into reflexivity (Giddens 1991). First of all, the development of the ultrasound technology makes routine ultrasound scans an increasingly elaborated control of the expected baby's normality. Second, these conditions shape the whole clinical situation. The examination is 'shown' on the screen through the whole encounter, and is therefore in a sense 'forced' on the parents. This process of visualization can evoke further parental questions about the development, well-being, and normality of the baby they actually see, as well as about the midwife's professional assessments and judgements.

Notes

1 There are various conceptions of when a baby comes into existence, conceptions that build on scientific explanations, ideological ideas or religious convictions. It is therefore reasonable that there are different ways of talking about the baby-to-be growing in the woman's uterus. In this chapter, I chose to use the terms 'the expected baby' or 'the baby-to-be'. When I quote the parents or the midwife I use the term they use themselves.
2 In Swedish maternity care, the father-to-be accompanies the woman to the routine ultrasound scan in the majority of cases.
3 There has been a considerable change in the use of the ultrasound scan in pregnancy since the technology was first introduced some 25 years ago. It was then used only in cases when a disease or malformation was suspected (Swedish Council on Technology Assessment in Health Care 1998). Today, all pregnant women are offered a routine ultrasound scan and 97 per cent accept this offer (Swedish Research Council 2001). Similar to other clinical practices, the ultrasound examination is evaluated and subject to technical development, which means that the use of this technology in clinical practice changes over time.
4 The routine ultrasound scan is part of the health surveillance of pregnant women in Swedish maternity care (Swedish National Board of Health and Welfare 1996), and generally carried out by midwives with a special training in ultrasonography. The pregnant woman is informed about the routine ultrasound examination during the registration visit at the maternity health care centre, and an appointment is booked. A short booklet is handed over, with information about the purpose of the ultrasound examination and what it is possible to see at the scan.
5 For an extended treatment of the phases and the structure of the encounter, see my doctoral dissertation (Jonsson 2004).

References

Adelswärd, V. and Sachs, L. (1996) 'The meaning of 6.8: numeracy and normality in health information', *Social Science and Medicine*, 43: 1179–87.

Baggens, C. (2002) 'Nurses' work with empowerment during encounters with families in child healthcare', *Critical Public Health*, 12: 351–63.

Bredmar, M. and Linell, P. (1999) 'Reconfirming normality: the constitution of reassurance in talks between midwives and expectant mothers', in S. Sarangi and C. Roberts (eds), *Talk, Work and Institutional Order*, Berlin: Mouton de Gruyter.

Draper, J. (2002) 'It was a real good show: the ultrasound scan, fathers and the power of visual knowledge', *Sociology of Health and Illness*, 24: 771–5.

Duden, B. (1993) *Disembodying Women*, London: Harvard University Press.

Drew, P. and Heritage, J. (eds) (1992) *Talk at Work*, Cambridge: Cambridge University Press.

Georges, E. (1996) 'Fetal ultrasound imaging and the production of authoritative knowledge in Greece', *Medical Anthropology Quarterly*, 10: 157–75.

Giddens, A. (1991) *Modernity and Self-Identity: Self and Society in the Late Modern Age*, Cambridge: Polity Press.

Green, J.M. (1994) 'Women's experiences of prenatal screening and diagnosis', in L. Abramsky and J. Chapple (eds), *Prenatal Diagnosis: The Human Side*, London: Chapman and Hall.

Hydén, L.C. and Mishler, E. (1999) 'Language and medicine', *Annual Review of Applied Linguistics*, 19: 174–92.

Jonsson, A.-C. (2004) 'Dokument inifrån. Ultraljudsbilder och visualisering av det väntade barnet' (Document from within: ultrasound images and visualization of the expected child), Dissertation. Linköping: Linköping Studies in Arts and Science, No 300 (in Swedish).

Lupton, D. (1999) 'Risk and the ontology of pregnant embodiment', in D. Lupton (ed.), *Risk and Sociocultural Theory: New Directions and Perspectives*, Cambridge: Cambridge University Press.

Mishler, E. (1984) *The Discourse of Medicine: Dialectics of Medical Interviews*, Norwood, NJ: Ablex.

Mitchell, L.M. and Georges, E. (1997) 'Cross-cultural cyborgs: Greek and Canadian women's discourses on fetal ultrasound', *Feminist Studies*, 23: 373–401.

Olin Lauritzen, S. and Sachs, L. (2001) 'Normality, risk and the future: implicit communication of threat in health surveillance', *Sociology of Health and Illness*, 23: 497–516.

Petchesky, R. (1987) 'Foetal images: the power of visual culture in the politics of reproduction', in M. Stanworth (ed.), *Reproductive Technologies: Gender, Motherhood and Medicine*, Cambridge: Polity Press.

Sandelowski, M. (1994) 'Channels of desire: fetal ultrasonography in two use-contexts', *Qualitative Health Research*, 4: 262–80.

Shilling, C. (1993) *The Body in Social Theory*, London: Sage.

Silverman, D. (1987) *Communication and Medical Practice*, London: Sage.

Strong, P. (1979) *The Ceremonial Order of the Clinic: Parents, Doctors and Medical Bureaucracies*, London: Routledge and Kegan Paul.

Swedish Council on Technology Assessment in Health Care (1998) *Rutinmässig ultraljudsundersökning under graviditeten* (Routine ultrasound screening during pregnancy), SBU-report nr 139, Stockholm (in Swedish).

Swedish National Board of Health and Welfare (1996) *Hälsovård före, under och efter graviditeten*, 1996: 7 (Healthcare before, during and after pregnancy), Stockholm: Socialstyrelsen (in Swedish).

Swedish Research Council (2001) *Tidig fosterdiagnostik. Konsensusuttalande* (Early foetal diagnosis), Stockholm: Swedish Research Council (in Swedish).

Turner, B.S. (1992) *Regulating Bodies: Essays in Medical Sociology*, London: Routledge.

Weir, L. (1998) 'Pregnancy ultrasound in maternal discourse', in Shildrick, M. and Price, J. (eds), *Vital Signs: Feminist Reconfigurations of the Bio/logical Body*, Edinburgh: Edinburgh University press.

Williams, S.J. (1997) 'Modern medicine and the uncertain body: from corporeality to hyperreality?', *Social Science and Medicine*, 45: 1041–9.

6   A normal pregnancy?

Women's experiences of being at high risk after ultrasound screening for Down syndrome

Sonja Olin Lauritzen,
Susanne Georgsson Öhman and
Sissel Saltvedt

Introduction

The development of medical technology in the field of reproductive health has been quite dramatic through recent decades. New technology has been developed, and also introduced into medical practice, making possible new types of assessments of deviance from normality. Some of these technologies, such as the ultrasound scan, have been turned into routine tests in clinical practice. Today, the ultrasound scan is part of health surveillance of pregnant women in most high-income countries. It was first introduced as a method to provide information of importance for a safe delivery,[1] but the ultrasound technology has gradually become more sophisticated and it is now possible to detect an increasing range of foetal abnormalities, even earlier in pregnancy. One of the recent developments in this direction, that we will address in this chapter, is nuchal translucency screening at ultrasound examination for early detection of Down syndrome (Snijders *et al.* 1998). Nuchal translucency screening is currently being tested and evaluated in Sweden as well as in other countries, and discussed as a possible new routine method to be included in national programmes of health surveillance of all pregnant women.[2]

The development of the new ultrasound screening for Down syndrome, as do other technologies to detect foetal abnormality, raises a series of psychological and ethical questions (Williams *et al.* 2002; see also Chapter 4 in this volume) as well as questions concerning the social impact of this screening, some of which we want to address in this chapter. From a sociological point of view, the ultrasound screening, targeting all pregnant women, can be discussed and problematized as an exponent of 'surveillance medicine' (Armstrong 1995). Of particular interest is the shift in the medical gaze inherent in this paradigm, from the actual to the potential presence of disease or disability, and thus a focus on early detection of deviance from normality. This shift, and the increasing medical-technological possibilities to detect abnormality, has been discussed as contributing to a wider shift in the relationship between lay people and medicine (de Swaan 1990). Screening for a particular abnormality confronts people with 'a small risk of a great misfortune' (ibid.) in those who see themselves as healthy. Even simply belonging to a population, such as pregnant women, will in this sense offer a status of 'being-at-risk' (Lupton 1995; Scott *et al.* 2005). As the development of new medical technology continuously adds new possibilities to detect deviance at an early stage, new states of 'being-at-risk' are being created. This, in turn, raises questions about the meaning of the status of being-at-risk for those who are subject to screening.

For the individual, screening seems to enhance an uncertainty about health and normality, an uncertainty that goes beyond test results that confirm normality (Davison *et al.* 1994). Earlier studies of various types of screening have shown how people struggle to understand the outcome of screening tests, often presented as a figure or a chart, and also how they try to make sense of these outcomes in the context of their life-worlds (Parsons and Atkinson 1992). Just being subject to screening can evoke uncertainty in the individual, even when no deviance is found (Adelswärd and Sachs 1996; Olin Lauritzen and Sachs 2001). Of particular interest is how people with not normal outcomes are placed in a liminal zone, 'between and betwixt' health and illness, as they wait for definite results (Forss *et al.* 2004; Scott *et al.* 2005) and how anxiety and worries can remain even after confirmation of normal results (Green 1990; Statham 1993; Santalahti 1996).

The ultrasound scan, as such, is something that pregnant women[3] as well as the population in general nowadays are familiar with and take for granted as part of maternity health care.[4] The offer to have an ultrasound scan is not often refused (Swedish Council on Technology Assessment in Health Care 1998). One central feature of the ultrasound scan is that it visualizes the inner body of the pregnant woman and makes the foetus the object of a medical as well as parental 'gaze'. As Ann-Cristine Jonsson points out in Chapter 5 in this volume, the image of the expected baby produced by the ultrasound technology is seen and interpreted from a professional as well as parental perspective at the ultrasound examination, and typically commented on from both perspectives in terms of the normality of the baby. Previous studies of parents' experiences of the routine ultrasound scan have shown that the scan is understood primarily as a routine test to confirm normality and as a social event when they are given the opportunity to see the baby for the first time (Sandelowski 1994; Baillie *et al.* 2000). For many parents-to-be, the ultrasound scan has such an important confirmative role that they wait until after the examination before announcing the pregnancy (Eklin *et al.* 2004). However, they are not always aware of the medical purpose of the examination (Marteau 1995; Al-Jader *et al.* 2000; Garcia *et al.* 2002).

Ultrasound screening for Down syndrome, however, is a technology that is new in several ways. First, it makes possible a new type of screening of the foetus, that is to detect foetuses with an increased risk of Down syndrome.

Second, this ultrasound screening is carried out in the first trimester of the pregnancy (gestational week 10–14), and thus intervenes in the life of the pregnant women at an earlier stage of pregnancy than methods previously used. As Statham *et al.* (1997) among others have argued, women's reactions to pre-natal screening have to be understood within the context of the psychology associated with pregnancy itself. Particularly the first and last trimesters of the pregnancy are characterized by an increased sensitivity and anxiety. Third, in contrast to other screening targets, this chromosomal abnormality has no other 'treatment' than selective abortion, and not all women will consider a termination of the pregnancy as an option (Delholm and Olsen 1992; Tymstra 1991).

In the exploration of the social impact of a new type of screening, it is important to take account also of the social context of this screening. A special feature of the ultrasound screening for Down syndrome is that it is carried out within the context of the well-established and familiar maternity health care services for all pregnant women, services that have a range of tasks aiming at promotion of health and normality. Within this programme, pregnant women will be offered various examinations and assessments of their health, and the health of the foetus, as well as psycho-social support and health educational sessions. This programme of maternity health care seems to be understood by Swedish parents mainly as a means to check that everything *is* 'okay' (Bredmar and Linell 1999; Olin Lauritzen and Sachs 2001).

The individual pregnant woman of course brings her own expectations and embodied experiences[5] to these encounters with the maternity services, experiences that will guide her also if the assessments that are carried out, explicitly or implicitly, 'question' the normality of the baby she is expecting. These expectations will have to be understood also against the back-drop of the way pregnancy in Western culture is understood to be part of ordinary life, constantly referred to as normal or natural (also in conversations between midwives and pregnant women, see Bredmar and Linell 1999), albeit a unique and significant experience in the life of the individual woman.

The screening for Down syndrome is thus part of an ultrasound examination, and ultrasound examinations are primarily understood as confirmation of normality and as a social event. The ultrasound examination is in turn embedded in the well-established and 'supportive' maternity health care services. As pointed out by Press and Browner (1997), broad patient acceptance of a new form of prenatal screening can be accomplished 'under the rubric of an older, and non-controversial, medical practice – routine prenatal care' (1997: 987). Here, we want to explore the meaning and significance of screening for Down syndrome within the everyday life of the woman, by looking further into women's experiences of the situation they find themselves in when normality is questioned after ultrasound screening for Down syndrome in early pregnancy.

Nuchal translucency screening for Down syndrome

In Sweden, as in many other countries, pregnant women are currently offered a routine ultrasound scan in the second trimester, and this offer is accepted by a vast majority (97 per cent according to national statistics). Women aged over 35 are counselled about their risk of carrying a foetus with Down syndrome on the basis of their age and are offered an invasive test to examine the foetus, the rationale being that the risk of giving birth to a baby with Down syndrome increases with maternal age. During the last decade, medical research has established that there is a strong association between an increased space of fluid that can be measured at an ultrasound examination carried out in gestational weeks 10–14, and Down syndrome. Drawing on this association, a new non-invasive technique for assessing the risk for Down syndrome has been developed: nuchal translucency screening by means of an ultrasound examination (Saltvedt *et al.* 2005).

A fluid-filled space at the back of the foetal neck (nuchal translucency), which exists only in early pregnancy, is measured in millimetres. Using software, a risk score is estimated based on this measurement in combination with maternal age and length of gestation. The main purpose is thus to identify women at high risk of carrying a baby with Down syndrome, and to offer these women an invasive test for foetal karyotyping to confirm or dismiss a Down syndrome diagnosis. The rational for introducing the nuchal translucency method is that this method will be more efficient in predicting risk for Down syndrome than the current practice based on maternal age. This can in turn reduce the total number of invasive tests that have to be carried out to confirm chromosomal abnormality, tests that are not unproblematic as they also cause a certain number of miscarriages.

As this ultrasound screening is still fairly new, women's experiences have not yet been studied to any great extent. A survey that was part of a randomized controlled trial in Sweden indicated that just taking part in the ultrasound screening did not cause more disturbed emotional well-being or worry about the baby's health than a routine scan (Georgsson Öhman *et al.* 2004). However, some in-depth qualitative studies of psychological reactions in women who received false positive results (indicating chromosomal abnormality) showed that these women expressed strong feelings of anxiety, which for some also lasted after confirmation of normality and after the birth of a healthy baby (Baillie *et al.* 2000; Georgsson Öhman *et al.* 2006).

The case of false positive screening results is an inevitable part of all screening procedures, an outcome that will question normality in a more direct way and take on particular importance (Davison *et al.* 1994). In this chapter, we will explore pregnant women's understanding of false positive screening results, more specifically women's ways of understanding information about being at high risk of carrying a foetus with Down syndrome after ultrasound screening. We will draw on interviews with 20 women[6] who received a high risk result at the ultrasound scan, in this study defined as a risk of 1:250 or higher, but in whom the invasive test results later revealed normal foetal chromosomes. After the high risk information, the women were offered an invasive test to confirm or dismiss a Down syndrome diagnosis. When the results from the invasive tests were confirmed as negative (no indication of Down syndrome) approximately four weeks after the scan, they were also offered a follow-up ultrasound scan in gestational week 18–20. The women were recruited consecutively from those who received high risk results in a trial of foetal screening in the Stockholm region in 1999–2002 (Georgsson Öhman *et al.* 2006). They were between 23 and 42 years old, expecting their first or second child, and had risk scores ranging between 1:20 and 1:250. Six of the women who were older than 35 received risk scores that in effect were not higher than their age-related risk.

The women were interviewed, in their homes, on three occasions: first after the early ultrasound scan and the risk information, secondly after the invasive test and confirmation of normality and finally two months after the birth of a healthy baby.[7] The interviews are seen as stories told by the women about their experiences of the ultrasound screening and the period following the high risk information, where the women also had the opportunity to add new experiences and retrospective reflections through the follow-up interviews. In this chapter, the focus is on how the women try to make sense of their experiences and how issues of normality and deviance (of the baby as well as the pregnancy) surface in this process. Here, certain themes seem to be of particular interest: (1) the way the women account for their understanding of the risk score: what is a high, low or 'normal' risk, how the risk score is calculated and how it can be made more concrete; (2) the women's reflections on the normality of the baby, and also on their difficulties in thinking 'rationally' about the baby; (3) the meaning of the high risk information and re-evaluations of this information after the healthy baby is born.

Understandings of a high risk score

Generally, the women said they had looked forward to the ultrasound examination, and described their experiences of the scan, as such, in positive terms, although a few had been worried about something being wrong with the baby even before the scan. When talking about their reactions to the high risk information that they received after the scan, the six women who were older than 35 years described the high risk information as more or less in line with what they had expected, or not worse. When the remaining 14 women talked about their first reactions to the high risk score, they all used expressions describing something unexpected and shocking: 'it was a shock', 'tragic', 'everything became dark' it was 'a slap in the face'. Many of them described the period after being given the information as 'a vacuum' and that they took 'time-out' from the pregnancy while waiting for the results from the invasive test. This 'withholding' of the pregnancy, which we have described elsewhere (Georgsson Öhman *et al.* 2006) has also been shown in some of the few other studies so far carried out on women's reactions to ultrasound screening for Down syndrome. Women who were informed about a high risk score after ultrasound screening described feelings of anxiety and the ways they took 'time-out' and also residual feelings of anxiety even after confirmation of a normal result (Baillie *et al.* 2000).

Here, we first want to look in more detail at how the women try to make sense of the high risk information. All the women talked elaborately about how they tried to understand the risk score, the figure that was presented to them by the midwife, and came back to this issue through the three interviews. The analysis reveals some typical ways this is done: the women try to understand the figure as high or low, as compared with other risk scores and by trying to understand the figure in the context of how it is calculated. The women also try to understand the figure (and the risk), by comparing the figure with other figures, such as risk expressed in per cent, by visualizing the risk score and by comparing themselves with other women with different risk scores. In this process, different words are used, such as 'figure', 'risk score', 'chance', 'probability' and 'risk'. The women often oscillate between these different ways of trying to understand the risk score – intertwined with evaluations of how the information about the risk score was presented to them and also implications of the risk score in the context of their own lives. The character of the women's accounts can be illustrated by this first example from an interview with Ann, aged 30, who had a risk score of 1:208:

ANN: She did the measurements, and we watched and so on, and when it was all done and we had our pictures (the paper copies of the ultrasound picture), we looked at the risk profile that she had on a piece of paper, and at that point I was completely unprepared that something like this could happen. The thought hadn't crossed my mind, in fact. So I was quite, I mean shocked is a strong word, but I was very, very surprised that this would happen to me. Somehow, I had never been near the thought that it could happen, so I was very sad, I thought it was terrible, because when she explained, in a very good way, that it was a very small risk, it was a 0.5 per cent chance, and you can have an invasive test, right then, it felt like a fifty–fifty chance, it was so tragic, I thought, terrible. When we first saw those papers we didn't understand anything about the meaning of those figures, and then she explained that she had measured, measured the neck, she had measured the back and somehow multiplied with my age, the age of the foetus and come up with this risk that means 0.5 per cent probability that something is wrong. So I think she was very nice and calm. But of course we started to raise a lot of questions. What is the most common, and how big does the risk have to be to be dangerous and things like that, and I think she did it very well because she didn't give any direct answers, of course there aren't, but we very much wanted a figure, and she was fairly vague, but said, well the normal is approximately 1 to 600, but varies a lot. Because I think that otherwise you could easily have a hang up on figures and just see everything as a number, but now, it was more like us understanding that okay, it can happen and it can not happen and this depends on a lot of reasons that you cannot always understand. So I think she did it very well.

INTERVIEWER: How did you think about the figure, was it high or low?

ANN: Well first I thought it wasn't so high, one chance on 208, I thought that sounded little. But then, when she said that the average was 1 to 600 at my age, then I realized that I had a probability that was three times as high, ehh and then when I talked to a friend, who had also done this and had one chance on 3,000, then I felt like, goodness, what an enormous risk I have compared to, ehh, so it is so strange because it is so relative, but at the same time it could have said 1 to 20 I suppose, or 1 to 50, so thinking more pragmatically it feels as if 0.5 per cent probability is fairly little. And if it concerned anything else, if somebody told me there is a 0.5 per cent probability that you will miss your plane tomorrow, then I would have said, okay, my God, how good that I will not miss the plane. But when it comes to something important like this, it feels as [sigh] why couldn't it have been 0.05 or something like that, because it is so important.

We can see that Ann is first of all expressing her strong feelings of being surprised, it had never crossed her mind that she could be at risk, and her emotional reactions of sadness. She is trying to understand the risk score as high or low when reflecting on the risk figure, 208, also talking about this in per cent and even as a fifty–fifty chance. She compares the figure with the average for women her age as well as with the risk score of another woman she knows. In doing this, she oscillates between talking about the risk as low and high. She also comments on the midwife and the way she presented the information about the risk score as being very good. The high risk message was terrible, but the midwife was nice. Finally, she concludes that she wished it was lower, because this particular situation, expecting a baby, is so important, not a trivial thing such as missing a plane. This example illuminates the way the women in their accounts move between different ways of making sense of the high risk information, which we will look at in more detail in the next sections.

The risk score as high or low

All women talked about *how difficult* it was to understand the risk score. Particularly the younger women, under 35, said they could not remember that they had ever received any information beforehand about the risk assessment, and were somehow taken by surprise. (Albeit all the women had been informed as part of the research project.) The woman in the following example argues that she was not aware that she was going to receive any risk information immediately after the scan:

CECILIA: (28, risk score 1:227) I can't remember that anybody told me that I was going to get this kind of a high risk or low risk figure at once, right there, or what it could mean and in what way I could proceed afterwards depending on the information we had, so I was quite taken, neither Henrik or myself were quite prepared, even if it was not a catastrophe or anything.

Also, the high risk information was difficult to understand, in the sense of actually catching what the midwife was saying. Some women argued that even if they could hear what the midwife was saying, it was still difficult to understand the meaning of the high risk information. What did chromosome abnormality actually mean? The relationship to Down syndrome was not always clear. For instance, Cecilia said that she did not know if the chromosome abnormality could affect the baby in other ways, and she felt 'very stupid'. Even if most women seemed to know that the midwife would calculate a risk score based on measurements of the neck of the foetus and the mother's age, this still did not make it easy to understand:

BEATRICE: (32, risk score 1:219) I knew she was going to calculate, and she explained very well, I think, very clearly how it is done. I don't remember exactly how they do it, but it is something about the neck and my own age and, but ... I think that was very clear and easy to understand, but then there isn't much more you know, as it is an examination, exactly what it depends on, that is a bit difficult to understand.

The issue of the risk score as high or low emerges in all interviews. Typically, a first reaction to the risk score in itself, as either low or high, is followed by a re-interpretation where for example the low is understood as high or vice versa. In their accounts, most of the women *move back and forth* between talking about *the risk as high or low*. Daniela, 26, says 'So even if I had a risk factor of 1:238, it became something very big, even if it perhaps wasn't so big. Others have even higher risk factors, more to worry about'. She goes on to say 'The risk could have been bigger, it could have been 1:20 or 1:4 or whatever, but now it is 1:238, and that is a small risk even if it is a risk'. In the following example, it becomes even more clear how Beatrice moves back and forth between seeing the risk as high or low:

BEATRICE: (32, risk score 1:219) And then it was difficult to understand, even if it is called a high risk, it isn't actually a very high risk. I ended up on 1 to 219, but as it is called a high risk, it feels as if ohh, this is a high risk, but it is actually not such a high risk (Later Beatrice continues:) I have been thinking about that this is more difficult that it actually is, these risks of 1 to 200, I haven't quite understood how big the risks are, or how small. Probably it is fairly small but you think it is much, much bigger.

When they try to understand the risk score, the women also *ask for more information*, particularly information about how the risk score is *calculated*. For example, some women ask where 'the borders' are, indicating that they try to understand the possible range of outcomes. They also wonder how *the divide* is made between the high and low risk, for instance what it actually means that you are in the high risk zone if you have a risk of 1:249, but in a low risk zone if you have 1:251. One needs something to relate the risk figure to:

INTERVIEWER: You think it is difficult to use these figures
METTE: (29, risk score 1:71) Yes, I mean, 1 to 71 doesn't say very much. You want to know, what is the range that most women my age will find themselves in. Do I have an unreasonably high risk, or is it evenly spread on everybody from 1 to 250 and downwards, or have I ended up in the bunch where most women are, or, I still don't know actually (...) I think it is good to have a concrete information if the person you are talking to still understands it is statistics. I do understand that it is not exactly 1 to 71, that I can understand (...) but low and medium, I think you will get these question independently of how the information is presented
INTERVIEWER: Should one ask *how* low risk?
METTE: I do think they present these figures quite well, but you need something to relate them to.

Here, we can see that Mette wants to know what 'the range' for women her age is, that is what would be normal for women her age, or for 'most' women, again indicating an effort to relate the figure to something. The women ask what risk scores are possible, and what do other women have. 'Can they have one to two thousand?' They also wonder what 'the scale' is, and what the risk figure would be in per cent? One woman says that in the conversation with the midwife, her husband 'who thinks fast' said that their risk score of 1:227 is less than 0.05 per cent risk, and that is nothing. Also, the women try to *compare* their figure with other figures. Some compare with figures their pregnant friends or colleagues have received, but if the figures of their friends were much lower, they would feel even more at risk themselves. In the next example, Daniela argues that it would be easier for her if she had been able to compare with risk scores in her earlier pregnancies:

DANIELA: (26, risk score 1:238) It is so difficult, because if I had had something to compare with, if I had had these estimates with the two others as well, I would have had something to compare with. Now I just have this 1 to 238 that is circulating in my head, and I have nothing to relate to. If I had had it with the two others, I would have known that I had two healthy children even with the risk figure.

Understanding the risk score as high or low is obviously difficult, just reflecting on the figure per se. The women also give numerous examples of how they saw this difficulty as related to the situation they found themselves in. Some described that they were in 'a shock', or that they became very sad and cried, and therefore did not catch so much of the information. Others said that they could suddenly feel that the risk, which was not so high, suddenly was a very big risk after all, relating this 'change' to their emotional state.

When the women account for their experiences of the high risk information, one characteristic pattern is that they also reflect on the ways they 'think'; how difficult it is to integrate or absorb the information, or think 'rationally'; how they try to think in a certain way, for example to think 'positively' or to think about the baby as healthy. In the following example, the woman talks about her difficulties in understanding the high risk information.

METTE: (29, risk score 1:71) The midwife didn't say very much. She told me about the statistics and about the routines they follow, but she didn't say very much more and that was good because I wasn't able to absorb anything more. I was too much in a shock, I wouldn't have been able to understand any more information right then (...) I don't think statistics is difficult, but when it comes to yourself, it is very difficult to put it into a rational context, I think.

Mette argues that it was difficult for her to 'absorb' the information, and she relates this to herself in the particular situation, 'right then' referring to when the midwife gave her the high risk information. Interestingly, she does not find the statistics, the figure, difficult. The difficulties have to do with herself and the state she is in. These types of reflections on their own, *difficulties to think in a clear way* or to think *rationally*, as they say, are typical of the way the women talk about their experiences. Understanding the risk score as high or low is thus not straightforward, and the women elaborately describe their own efforts to understand what it means and the various ways they try to contextualize the risk score.

Belonging to a high risk group

Another way of reflecting on the risk score is to focus on the fact that when the risk is one to something, *somebody has to be the one*. Even if it is a small risk, somebody has to be the one that is not normal:

DANIELA: (26, risk score 1:238) Well, at the same time as it is a very small risk, it is after all 238, 237 of 238 are healthy, but still I think that somebody has to be this one, and that could just as well be my baby. Of course it would have been even worse if it had been 1 to 40 or 1 to 20 or less, but still, it somehow echoes in my head that the risk is there, the risk you wouldn't have believed existed.

When talking about the difficulties in understanding the high risk information, Daniela returns several times to the fact that she had not expected to be at risk. She is young, 26, and has already given birth to two healthy babies and thought that having this baby was going to be just as easy as the other two. Of course, the thought that something could be wrong was always there, also with the earlier babies, but not that she could be in a 'risk zone'. 'It became much more'. Being in a 'risk zone' is something that also other women talk about. Beatrice says she knew that they were going to calculate which risk zone she would belong to:

BEATRICE: (32, risk score 1:219) I asked how high is this risk, and then she (the midwife) made a circle on a piece of paper, like this, and all those with a high risk around 300, she placed in a small circle in the middle, which I belonged to, and then I understood that even if the risk is not so high, you belong to a group with a higher risk than the average, and that is a little difficult to understand with all the figures and so on.

To Beatrice, the high risk score means that she belongs to a risk group, a certain group of women, and this understanding seems to be supported by the way the high risk women are placed in 'a circle in the middle' by the midwife as she tries to visualize the risk. Also in the next example, the woman talks about herself as belonging to a risk group.

INTERVIEWER: What did you find out, what did they say?
JENNY: (32, risk score 1:250) That I belonged to a risk group, that there was a one to 250 chance that it would be, well that the baby would have chromosome abnormalities [cries] in a way it is not a great chance, but I still think it felt [cries] as if, yes as if it was almost a clear information about something being wrong, that's how I experienced it, but you don't think quite logically somehow [cries] (...) she (the midwife) wasn't actually in doubt about the figure, she thought she had very clear results of the measurements, so there was nothing to discuss. But still, she tried to say, think about that 249 will be healthy and the chance is really not very big, and things like that, to make me not break down completely.

Again, characteristic of the women's accounts is that they argue that they *want to think in a certain way*. By many, this is expressed as 'thinking positively'. Opposite to the arguments about being the 'one' that we have seen earlier, Jenny argues that she wants to 'think positively' by thinking that she is *not* 'the one', but one of the 249 that are fine.

JENNY: (32, risk score 1:250) I try to think about that 249 will be fine, and that I will be one of them. And she said that 1 per cent of all pregnancies will anyway not go well, because I asked about the risk related to the invasive test, which is 1 to 100, so in fact that chance of something going wrong is bigger. So that is how I will think, then it will be a bit more positive. But things go up and down, very much so. You should try not to think so much, but that is very difficult.

Jenny says that when she waited for the results from the invasive test, every second day she thought that something was wrong, 'but somehow I have to think positively, or I will drive myself crazy'. She also tries to think about the fact that there is anyway always a risk that something will go wrong. The chance of something going wrong with the invasive test, for instance, is 1:100. 'I just have to think like that, I can't think just negatively'. But there are difficulties in doing this. She puts it down to herself: 'then I think it is me, I just have to think like that'. In the end, Jenny says, she tries *not* to think.

Seeing oneself as belonging to, or being placed in, a risk group is thus a way to understand the high risk information. Another illustrative example is Jenny, who comments on her own risk score of 1:250, on the border of having a high risk outcome, as being 'the last, I just slipped in'. Ending up in a risk group means that something is demanded from you, you have to take certain decisions. This notion of a risk group seems to be supported by the ways the women try to understand the risk information by making it more concrete or visual, frequently referring to the midwife's efforts to explain the high risk information.

Trying to visualize the risk

The women thus talk about the midwife and how she tries to help them to understand the risk score. One way is to *make the risk score more visual*. Again, the risk score is difficult to understand, as Beatrice argues, particularly when you have to 'take a decision based on something you don't understand'. She describes how she tries to understand better by visualizing her risk of 1:219, to create an image of the risk. She refers to what the midwife told her about how she could make the risk score more concrete:

BEATRICE: (32, risk score 1:219) Imagine that you give birth to 219 babies, if you would have 219 babies, one of them would have this deviance. The risk is that you think about 219 mothers with babies in the street, so one of these babies would be, but that is not the case, you must not think like that, because that is wrong, it's supposed to be that if every individual gives birth to that number of babies, one of them will be born with, so I have tried to think more like that, or if you try to think of 219 things in front of you, you can count paving-stones in the street or something and try to understand. I guess that image of the 219 is easier to understand than looking at a figure on a piece of paper. And this risk is so small, it is so small that you could hardly, if you think about the risk of a miscarriage before the twelfth week, that's 15 per cent, so that risk is incredibly higher than this risk, and if you have gotten past that risk, then you feel there shouldn't be any great problems to get past this second risk which is much smaller. But as it is called high risk, it is difficult to think, well [sigh].

As we see here, Beatrice tries to think of an image that will make 219 more visual and thus more concrete, something that will be more easy to understand than a figure on a piece of paper. She also compares her risk figure with another risk that is known to her, the risk of a miscarriage in early pregnancy. This other risk is expressed in per cent 'that's 15 per cent' and she draws the conclusion that this is a much higher risk than the ultrasound risk score of 1:219. She continues to relate these two risk figures to each other by saying that once you have gotten past the first higher one, there shouldn't be any great problems getting past the second and smaller one. Also in the following example we see how the woman tries to compare her risk score with other risk estimates in pregnancy:

METTE: (29, risk score 1:71) I had nothing to relate these figures to, and then I thought it was very much. I also asked about the invasive test, how big is the risk for a miscarriage. That risk is somewhere between 0.5 per cent and 1 per cent. Then we can say 1 to 150, and then this feels like a big risk too. But if you imagine that you line up 71 women and just one, then it feels a bit less, but I, those figures became very big, to me it was a very big risk.

What we see here, is that the women in their accounts vividly describe their difficulties in understanding the meaning of the risk score, and the various methods they try to use. They do try to understand better by contextualizing, comparing and visualizing the risk figure. In doing this, they are looking for something to hold on to. They draw on notions of normality to create a frame of reference. They reflect on what can be expected and what is normal. 'What is normal risk for me or for a woman my age?' They also position themselves within or outside normality, as belonging to or not belonging to a high risk group. Also, importantly, the women compare their risk figures with other risks, or rather implications of risks, that they see as trivial (such as missing a plane).

The women under 35 did not expect a risk of chromosomal abnormality from the ultrasound scan, they were 'taken by surprise', which can be understood against the backdrop of cultural understandings of the scan as a 'routine' procedure in antenatal care (which of course raises problems concerning informed consent). They struggle to understand the high risk information, and try to grasp the risk figure they are given as high or low by inquiring into how the figure is calculated and the divide between the normal and the not normal. But most of all they try to understand the risk by making it more concrete and possible to compare with other phenomena or situations in their life-worlds. Similar 'strategies' to understand risk information have been demonstrated in other studies of screening or genetic predictive testing where people are presented with a risk figure (Parsons and Atkinson 1992; Adelswärd and Sachs 1996; Olin Lauritzen and Sachs 2001). Here, however, the risk figure is not related to the bodies of those receiving the information, as in most types of screening, but to the baby they are carrying. The women's elaborate accounts of the difficulties in understanding the risk score, and as they say 'thinking rationally', can also be understood within the context of the early phase of the pregnancy they are in, when the baby is something 'new' that has to be understood and integrated into their lives.

Thinking about the baby as normal

As we have seen, the women reflect on their own thinking concerning the risk score. They try to think in a particular way, for instance to think positively, or they try not to think, which is also typical for how they talk about the baby. Here, different patterns can be found in the material. Some women talk more elaborately about how they try hard to think 'positively', to *think about the baby as healthy*, others talk about not being able to think anything else than about the baby as *ill or disabled*. The women also argue that they try *not* to think at all. Typically, the women oscillate between different future scenarios, of becoming a mother of a healthy child or a child with Down syndrome, including also the scenario of a termination of the pregnancy.

Trying to sustain an image of a healthy baby

The 'positive' thinking could for instance be expressed as wishing they could think about the image from the ultrasound scan as a healthy baby. We will here look into the case of Cecilia (aged 28, risk score 1:227) to illustrate this line of argument. Cecilia wishes she could think 'of the lovely brain and everything that looked so good' at the ultrasound examination. But this is not so easy. Unfortunately she thinks more about the information she and her husband had, and all the images of children that passed through her head, or of 'how I as a parent am going to cope with the situation if it is a Down syndrome and what it means'. She oscillates between thinking of the baby as healthy and as a baby with Down syndrome:

CECILIA: Some days I am completely convinced that we will have a healthy baby, and then other days I think, my God, how is a child with Down syndrome going to cope with life in our society that is so individualistic, and how am I as a parent, or we as parents, going to cope with a child that will always be a child, even as grown up, that frightens me more, children will always demand a lot of time and presence from their parents, but as grown up they will be independent, but I am not sure a child with Down's syndrome will ever. It is these thoughts I have had (...) At the same time I think that if anybody should have such a baby, it should be Henrik and me, we are so confident persons, I think we would deal with it very well and I am sure that such a child would bring a lot of happiness, so you can twist it back and forth (...) I think that independently of what happens, it is as I said very good to find out and to have these thoughts already now (Interview 1)

After the risk of chromosome abnormality is confirmed to be false, and after the follow-up scan, the images of the baby can be re-assessed. Also, the baby is now bigger and has a more baby-like look:

CECILIA: The body proportions looked better now, before (at the first scan) the head was so enormously big, it looked a bit strange, but now, it looked like a baby and it was nicer to look at than the first time, because now you really saw the little fingers clearly, everything was more clear, and then I had this feeling of being proud, how wonderful, just imagine that this is our baby, and it looks really healthy (laughter) you could see the brain so clearly and the heart, yes it was fascinating (Interview 2).

Here, in the second interview after the invasive test and follow-up scan, the risk of Down syndrome has been dismissed. Cecilia talks about how the baby looks at the follow-up scan. She can see the body parts very clearly and she says that the baby is 'really healthy' and it is all wonderful and fascinating. Having said this, Cecilia goes on to say that independently of the results, it would have been fine. Even if the baby had Down syndrome, she and her husband would want the baby and love it just as much, 'even if it is not quite healthy, if you think in a scale of normality'.

Thinking of the baby as ill or disabled

Others describe how they have not being able to think about the baby as healthy or well, even if they try to. They can only think about the baby as ill. Mette, aged 29, with a risk score of 1:71 is one example:

METTE: My thoughts have been mixed. In my world, the baby was ill, that's how it was. I think I prepared myself much more for how an abortion would be, even if I hadn't made up my mind about having an abortion if the baby actually was ill, than actually feeling happy about the baby. I didn't. But I thought much more about it, both emotionally, how I would cope, and practically, how is it done, pain relief, going through labour, will I be able to look at the baby? Practical things, my thoughts were more focused on that (Interview 2).

Mette talks about how she thinks about her baby as definitely ill or disabled after the risk information. She also comments on her way of thinking, how her thoughts move from worries about the baby towards 'practical' issues concerning a possible abortion. She also comments that she knows that these thoughts are irrational, but argues that still, in 'her head', the baby is ill, and she sees the 'irrational thoughts' as dealing with the crisis ahead of her. Interestingly, she still thinks that her own body feels normal, 'like a normal pregnancy'. Even in the last interview, after her healthy baby is born, Mette talks about how during the pregnancy she saw the baby as 'just a swelling or something' that she just wanted to get 'over and done with'. She didn't think of it so much as a baby, or an individual. 'No, this pregnancy has just been long and difficult and I haven't been well, so I think I didn't feel so much worries for him being ill, I just wanted the pregnancy to come to an end'.

Trying not to think at all

Other women argue that they try to *not* think at all. In the following example, Ann, aged 30, risk score 1:208, talks about how, if everything had been fine, she would have looked a lot at the videotape from the first scan. After the risk information, she did not watch it at all because that would make her think about the baby, which she did not want to do:

ANN: If there hadn't been anything not quite right, I am sure I would have watched that film (the video from the ultrasound examination) at least 25 times by now, just because it would have been such fun to show everybody who visited, but now we haven't, not even once, it is just laying there on the shelf where we put it when we came home, and ever since we haven't looked at it because it would feel so strange to look at it now, I think, we just lost track and it is somehow, it is not so awful but it still feels as if, okay, maybe it is going to be a baby, maybe not, and I am fairly prepared for that, and that is the reason why I don't want to watch that film, it would just be a strange feeling
INTERVIEWER: In what way would it be a strange feeling?
ANN: Well, because then I would think even more, is there going to be a baby or maybe not, or, now he is laying there kicking and in a couple of months maybe he will not (Interview 1).

To Ann, it would be 'a strange feeling' to look at the video of the baby, as this would make her think even more about the baby as healthy or not.

She goes on to reflect that the baby may not even be alive in a couple of months. The 'strange feeling' can of course be understood as an expression of uncertainty if the face of these possibilities, or not wanting to become emotionally 'involved' with a baby that is maybe not going to be born. After the results from the invasive test, Ann speaks more explicitly about normality:

ANN: It was a very nice letter from the clinic, from that doctor, I don't remember his name, but the nice thing was that it said normal several times in bold letters, that it was a normal result and that it is completely normal. That was very considerate, I think. I gather it is a word that all parents want to hear all the time, that it is normal
INTERVIEWER: So that was what the test showed?
ANN: Yes, it was, one could see immediately that it was normal (Interview 2).

After the high risk information, the baby's normality is thus largely questioned by the women. Even those who try to think about the baby as healthy would typically oscillate between seeing the baby as healthy and ill or disabled. Furthermore, these reflections are extended into the baby as not being alive or into thinking about their baby as a Down syndrome child and what this would mean for the child, themselves as parents and for their whole family. The possibility that the baby, who is still in the womb, is not going to 'be there' in the near future is a line of thought that surfaces in various ways in many interviews, as we have already seen. This possibility is explicitly or implicitly related to a decision about an abortion, which might follow a Down syndrome diagnosis, or a miscarriage due to the invasive test or just something that could happen anyway. The women quite explicitly account for their images and fantasies of a baby with an abnormality. They think about the future, which might possibly be a life with a child that has Down syndrome, and what it could be like to parent such a child. They also go on to reflect on what life would be like, and the difficulties created by the mismatch between the needs of a family with a Down syndrome child and the attitudes and conditions in society at large.

Re-evaluations of the risk assessment after the birth

In the third and last interview, two months after the birth of a healthy baby, the women present a range of arguments why the risk assessment was something good or bad to have participated in. The good things were that if there is an abnormality, it is better to find out at an early stage, and also that going through this difficult process of risk assessment will make you even more happy if your baby turns out to be healthy and make you feel more 'humble' and grateful in the face of what life can bring. The negative things have to do with the fact that they had to go through a very difficult period while pregnant, that this in effect ruined that period and prevented them from feeling happiness and confidence as pregnant women. For some, such negative experiences loomed large even after the healthy baby was born.

Again, the women who tried to think 'positively' argued that the way the risk assessment made you think about parenthood and what parenthood can bring was a good thing. We will continue to follow Cecilia. In the first interview, she talks about the benefit of the ultrasound screening:

CECILIA: Somehow, I feel that if you have had the benefit of having this examination (the ultrasound scan) you should draw on it and go all the way, I think I feel that strongly, because otherwise there is no point in knowing that the risk for me is 1 to 227, but of course you can have different opinions, and I know that some people think it is awful to have an invasive test to somehow sort out if the baby is healthy or has a chromosomal abnormality, but Henrik and me, we think it is good to have that information and to be prepared (Interview 1).

There has to be a point in having the risk information, and one point is to make you, as a parent, prepared for whatever the future will bring. After the invasive test and confirmation of normality, she continues along the same line of argument. She is pleased that she was confronted with the 'more serious part' of being an expecting mother:

CECILIA: I think I would have lived in a 'tutti-frutti' world if I had not gone through this process (laughter) (…) there was more of a serious part, and I am still happy about that, now afterwards, I am happy that I had that period and realized that the responsibility, that parenthood will always demand something from you, that you can't just carry on and think that everything is fine (Interview 2).

Cecilia also thinks she is a more happy mother now, as compared with if she had not gone through the examination. She is happy that she had this experience, she learnt that 'a lot can happen in pregnancy' and also that you cannot take anything for granted. In the last interview she says:

CECILIA: I think I am more grateful for her being so fine. It is possible, but difficult to tell, it is possible that I would have been grateful even if I had not gone through this thing with the high risk group and those things, but I think it made us think about what life is and that you cannot take anything for granted (Interview 3).

She concludes that it was something positive to have had the ultrasound screening, even though she was still frustrated about not having understood more when she received the results, what it actually means to belong to a risk group. Also some of the parents that definitely thought that the baby was ill or not normal argued that it was a good thing to have the early information about a possible deviation. The good thing about finding out about deviance at an early stage is articulated by Ann:

ANN: After we had got over that it all was so sad, I think we somehow realized that it would be very good to find out if something was wrong, very good to find out early, I think we were lucky to be placed in the early group [to have the early ultrasound] so I think we, it was probably something unconscious that you try to turn it into something positive, but I think we succeeded very well in doing that, because suddenly we saw it as if we were lucky instead of unfortunate, as we thought at first when we saw the risk per cent (Interview 1).

If something should be wrong with the baby, it would be good to know in advance. This can make you more prepared. Here Ann reflects on the misfortune that is transformed into something positive. She and her husband could suddenly see themselves as lucky instead of unfortunate, as they did when they first saw the risk figure, and they succeeded well in doing this. It is not only good to know in advance. Ann goes on to say that she will be even more happy if the baby turns out to be healthy and normal, compared with a situation without the risk assessment. She thinks she will appreciate the baby even more, if things go well. Having a healthy baby is in itself absolutely fantastic, 'but I think I will be even a little bit more happy'. The difficult period, difficult at the time, she thinks will not be remembered:

ANN: I think Johan and myself felt that, my God, it was good that we did this test, it could have been something, now it wasn't, it is not a big deal to worry for a while, later on, you will hardly remember that it was difficult somehow. I know I felt so at the time, but now I cannot remember that it was so very difficult or that it took such a long time (no) that's how it is, you forget about the difficult things (Interview 2).

In a few cases however, the woman was not happy about having had the ultrasound screening and about her pregnancy. To Mette, the high risk score was a shock, completely unexpected, as she was not yet 30 years old. In the first interview she says:

METTE: After having done the scan, I actually think one ought to think about these thing before deciding on the ultrasound scan, really, but most women have a scan nowadays, at least all my friends, and they talk about it as if 'have you done your scan yet?' But you don't talk about what the scan is actually for, to find deviancies, and what you do with that information. I haven't thought about this until now. (And later in the same interview:) If I would do it again, yes I have also thought about that, and I think I would, but what I regret a little, as I mentioned before, is that I didn't think about the consequences, and I shouldn't have done that just before this happened but before I got pregnant in the first place. Why do we have a scan, why do we go through all of this (...) so I can regret that I didn't think more about the consequences (Interview 1).

In the second interview, Mette again talks about her experience of being in a 'vacuum', and how she thinks about the baby as definitely ill, or maybe even dead, before the invasive test. Also after the confirmation of normality she could not feel happy:

METTE: This has caused so much mental suffering, because unfortunately I haven't been feeling very well after this (...) I haven't been able to feel happy about my pregnancy, even though I feel that other people think I should be happy (Interview 2).

Again, Mette argues that, after having her experiences, she had not quite understood (nor did other people) that the scan is actually a way of finding deviancies. If she became pregnant again she would want to be much more prepared that things can happen, and will not always turn out the way you have planned. Reflecting on the months of the pregnancy, Mette talks about her feelings for the baby:

METTE: It was just like a swelling or something, I just wanted to get it over and done with, I didn't think of so much as a baby, an individual, I can't say that I had any feelings (...) no this pregnancy has just been so long and difficult and I was not well (Interview 3).

The decisions a woman has to take while pregnant are here placed within the context of motherhood or parenthood. As an expecting mother you have an obligation to think about the baby that you are carrying. The notion of hurting the baby in the womb is a theme that surfaces in several contexts through the three interviews. When having to take a decision about the invasive test after the high risk information, worries about actually causing a miscarriage by having the test are deeply troubling to many women. Also, you have to be a happy mother to give the baby a good 'environment'. If you are very unhappy or stressed, this could endanger the health and wellbeing of the baby in the womb. This all has to do with responsibility.

Discussion and concluding comments

In this study, we have addressed women's experiences of being at high risk for carrying a baby with Down syndrome. Here, our focus is on women's ways of accounting for their experiences and understandings as they are confronted with a questioning of the normality of their baby after ultrasound screening for Down syndrome, a question that eventually is found to be false. We particularly want to discuss some central themes that emerge in the analysis of the women's accounts.

First, as we have seen, the women found it difficult to understand the information on high risk and to transform a test result to the level of their own individual life. It was thus difficult to assimilate the result as normal or not normal, and the women tended to rather oscillate between the poles of the perceived dichotomy of normality and abnormality, or make the abnormality their hypothesis. These understandings are in line with how lay representations of risk have been described as binary, which has been discussed also in another study of nuchal translucency screening for Down syndrome (Baillie *et al.* 2000). We would argue that this screening for Down syndrome, however, confronts the women not only with risk information that is difficult to interpret, but also, and immediately, with the profound and difficult question of giving birth to a disabled child or terminating the pregnancy and what that would mean in the context of their family lives.

Second, the women describe a process that they go through, starting with the expectation of a normal pregnancy that is interrupted by the unexpected high risk information after the ultrasound screening. The high risk information introduces a sudden shift from a routine examination of a 'normal pregnancy' to a high risk pregnancy. The women have to make sense of this sudden shift, and struggle to understand and assimilate the meaning of the high risk information. In this process, various future scenarios emerge, scenarios that revolve around quite dramatic issues such as a termination of the pregnancy or a future life with a disabled child. The offer of this screening, similar to other offers of prenatal tests, forces the woman to reflect on the very concrete options of an abortion or a version of motherhood that she had not expected.

The sudden shift to a high risk pregnancy is followed by the process of trying to return to a normal pregnancy. After the invasive tests and confirmation of normality, some women re-assess the high risk information as something 'positive' that has made them feel even more humble and grateful for their healthy baby. To them, the relief after confirmation of normality is depicted as returning to a normal pregnancy and a motherhood that is even more valued. To others, the difficulties after the high risk information have remained, and they say that they have not been able to return to a normal pregnancy. The 'returning' to a normal pregnancy is thus a complex process, not easily accomplished by all women. Interestingly, the efforts to detect abnormality by screening for Down syndrome are basically not questioned in these women's stories. Even after the 'shock' of the high risk information, the difficulties in understanding the risk figure and reflections on quite difficult future scenarios – which turned out to be based on a false outcome – most, but not all, women still argue that it was a 'good thing' to have had this information. To talk about these difficult experiences as something 'good' can in more psychological terms be interpreted as a way to handle a dilemma: 'what is, must be best' (Porter and Macintyre 1984; Van

Teijlingen *et al.* 2003). These quite paradoxical accounts can however also be understood as reflecting the women's efforts to return to normality by re-evaluating the worrying risk information as something 'good' that could be integrated into the experience of their own pregnancy as, in the end, normal. It is also possible that the Down syndrome screening is imbued with meaning associated to routine antenatal care (just another test), and to an understanding of the advantages of this care more generally (such as the relationship to an empathic midwife), as discussed by Press and Browner (1997) in their study of another prenatal diagnostic test, the maternal serum alpha fetoprotein.

The initial sense of relief after confirmation of normality has in other studies of the psychological reactions in pregnant women been found to be followed by residual feelings of worry and continued fears of abnormality, and it has been pointed out that the longevity of these feelings are still not known (Baillie *et al.* 2000). From a psychological perspective, Marteau *et al.* (1992) discuss how residual anxiety could be attributed to a generalized anxiety, or heightened awareness that 'something' could go wrong. The difficulties in reversing the belief that something is wrong observed by Marteau *et al.* are thus in line with the observations in this study, that not all women can make the transition from a high risk pregnancy back to an 'expectant' state of pregnancy (ibid.).

Third, the women in this study account not only for understanding of risk scores but also how this risk is understood in the context of motherhood, more precisely in the context of the moral responsibility for another being. Of particular interest is how they in this process describe different scenarios: that of the expected baby as normal and healthy, of a termination of the pregnancy after confirmation of abnormality, as well as the scenario of a future life as the mother of a disabled child. The high risk information confronts the women with scenarios of the abnormal, and the decisions they will have to take themselves in the face of this information. For many of the women, this immediately triggers reflections on a future motherhood with a disabled child. As Rapp argues, offers of a prenatal diagnosis turn women into 'moral pioneers' (2000: 310) as they are forced into an engagement with 'disability consciousness'. The development of foetal diagnostic tests thus mean that expectant parents increasingly are faced with the responsibility of deciding whether to use tests to discover characteristics of their foetus, and if something is discovered, the difficulty of having to decide what to do. Shakespeare (2003: 203) points out that 'This adds to the stress and anxiety of pregnancy for everyone, not just the tiny proportion in whom a genetic condition is diagnosed'. In this context he argues that the condition of Down syndrome 'has moved from being an unfortunate piece of bad luck, to being a blameworthy failure of surveillance and control' (ibid.: 205). This also means that this reproductive technology not only opens the pregnant body to control, but also the expected baby to be 'chosen' (Williams 1997: 1045).

These findings reflect one of the tensions inherent in surveillance medicine (Armstrong 1995). On the one hand, efforts are made to reduce risk (by better and more efficient methods to detect those at risk) and on the other hand, the individual is given responsibility for her own health (by presenting screening results and leaving the decisions to be taken to the individual).

While the health professionals can be assisted by new reproductive technology, the information about normality and abnormality produced by these technologies can, as we have seen in this chapter, take on quite different meanings for the individual woman and confront her with the moral responsibility for the consequences of the screening. These discrepancies between the medical objectives and the women's expectations and experiences need to be taken into consideration.

Finally, new reproductive technology not only raises questions about the social 'costs' and 'benefits' of these technologies, but also 'opens up' to debate issues which formerly belonged to the realm of biological 'givens' (Williams 1997: 1045). As new reproductive technology is developed, and more diagnostic tests are added to the routine surveillance of pregnant women, further research is needed to understand not only the social impact of the single technology, but also how the totality of the tests that women will encounter through a pregnancy will influence notions of the normal pregnancy and the biological 'givens' in reproduction.

Acknowledgements

Economic funding for this study has been gratefully received from the Swedish Foundation for Health Care Sciences and Allergy Research (Vårdalstiftelsen), the Centre for Health Care Sciences at the Karolinska Institute, and the South General Hospital in Stockholm. The study has been approved by the Regional Research and Ethical Committee at the Karolinska Institute.

Notes

1 The current aim of the routine ultrasound examination is to estimate the gestational age, to localize the placenta, to screen for multiple pregnancy and to detect structural malformations (Swedish National Board of Health and Welfare 1996).
2 In several countries, an ultrasound scan at 11–14 weeks is already being introduced as a routine offer in addition to the traditional scan in mid-pregnancy.
3 Today, antenatal care, and particularly the ultrasound scan, involves both parents-to-be (see for example Chapter 5 in this volume, and Draper's study (2002) of fathers' experiences of the ultrasound scan). This chapter, however, is based on an interview study with pregnant women.
4 In Sweden, the ultrasound examination is usually performed by a midwife with special training in ultrasonography.
5 We see an embodied approach to reproductive technology as one important avenue in the exploration of women's experiences, however it is not elaborated

on in this chapter. See also Ettorre (2000) for a feminist embodied approach to reproductive technology.

6 For this interview study, all together 24 women were recruited consecutively at four ultrasound units in the Stockholm region from the group of women who received high risk results (1:250 or higher) in a randomized controlled trial of foetal screening including risk assessment for Down syndrome by measurement of nuchal translucency which was carried out as a multi-centre study of 39,572 women in Sweden from 1999 to 2002 (Saltvedt et al. 2005). After an invasive test (amniocentesis or in a few cases chorionic villious sampling), Down syndrome was confirmed in four of the 24 cases, and these women made the choice to terminate the pregnancy. For the remaining 20 women, the high risk information turned out to be false.

7 The interviews were carried out by Susanne Georgsson Öhman and Sissel Saltvedt, who have professional backgrounds as midwife and obstetrician respectively.

References

Adelswärd, V. and Sachs, L. (1996) 'The meaning of numeracy and normality in health information talks', Social Science and Medicine, 43: 1179–87.

Al-Jader, L.N., Parry-Langdon, N. and Smith, R.J. (2000) 'Survey of attitudes of pregnant women towards Down syndrome screening', Prenatal Diagnosis, 20: 23–9.

Armstrong, D. (1995) 'The rise of surveillance medicine', Sociology of Health and Illness, 18: 737–44.

Baillie, C., Smith, J., Hewison, J. and Mason, G. (2000) 'Ultrasound screening for chromosomal abnormality: women's reactions to false positive results', British Journal of Health Psychology, 5: 377–94.

Bredmar, M. and Linell, P. (1999) 'Reconfirming normality: the constitution of reassurance in talks between midwives and expectant mothers', in S. Sarangi and C. Roberts (eds) Talk, Work and Institutional Order: Discourse in Medical, Mediation and Management Settings, Berlin: Mouton de Gruyter.

Davison, C., Macintyre, S. and Smith, G.D. (1994) 'The potential social impact of predictive genetic testing for susceptibility to common chronic diseases: a review and proposed research agenda', Sociology of Health and Illness, 16: 340–71.

Delholm, G. and Olsen, J. (1992) 'Ethical and psychological aspects of screening', in C. Hugod and J. Fog (eds) Screening, Why, When and How, The National Board of Health, Denmark.

Draper, J. (2002) '"It was a real good show": the ultrasound scan, fathers and the power of visual knowledge', Sociology of Health and Illness, 24: 771–95.

Eklin, M., Crang-Svalenius, E. and Dykes, A.-K. (2004) 'A qualitative study of mothers' and fathers' experiences of routine ultrasound examination in Sweden', Midwifery, 20: 335–44.

Ettorre, E. (2000) 'Reproductive genetics, gender and the body: "Please doctor, may I have a normal baby?"', Sociology, 34: 403–20.

Forss, A., Tishelman, C., Widmark, C. and Sachs, L. (2004) 'Women's experiences of cervical cellular changes: an unintentional transition from health to liminality?' Sociology of Health and Illness, 26: 306–25.

Garcia, J., Bricker, L., Henderson, J. et al. (2002) 'Women's views of pregnancy ultrasound: a systematic review', Birth, 29: 225–50.

Georgsson Öhman, S., Saltvedt, S., Grünewald, C. and Waldenström, U. (2004) 'Does fetal screening affect women's worries about the health of their baby? A randomized controlled trial of ultrasound screening for Down syndrome versus routine ultrasound screening', *Acta Obstetricia Gynecologica Scandinavia*, 83: 634–40.

Georgsson Öhman, S., Saltvedt, S., Waldenström, U., Grünewald, C. and Olin Lauritzen, S. (2006) 'Pregnant women's responses to information about an increased risk of carrying a baby with Down syndrome', *Birth*, 33: 64–73.

Green, J.M. (1990) *Calming or Harming? A Critical Review of Psychological Effects of Fetal Diagnosis on Pregnant Women*, London: Galton Institute Occasional Papers, second series.

Lupton, D. (1995) *The Imperative of Health: Public Health and the Regulated Body*, London: Sage.

Marteau, T.M. (1995) 'Towards informed decisions about prenatal testing: a review', *Prenatal Diagnosis*, 15: 1215–26.

Marteau, T.M., Cook, R., Kidd, J., Michi, S., Johnston, M., Slack, J. and Shaw, R. (1992) 'The psychological effects of false-positive results in prenatal screening for fetal abnormality: a prospective study', *Prenatal Diagnosis*, 12: 205–14.

Olin Lauritzen, S. and Sachs, L. (2001) 'Normality, risk and the future: implicit communication of threat in health surveillance', *Sociology of Health and Illness*, 23: 497–516.

Parsons, E. and Atkinson, P. (1992) 'Lay construction of genetic risk', *Sociology of Health and Illness*, 14: 437–55.

Porter, M. and Macintyre, S. (1984) 'What is, must be best: a research note on conservative or deferential responses to antenatal care provision', *Social Science and Medicine*, 19: 1197–200.

Press, N. and Browner, C.H. (1997) 'Why women say yes to prenatal diagnosis', *Social Science and Medicine*, 45: 979–89.

Rapp, R. (2000) *Testing Women, Testing the Fetus: The Social Impact of Amniocentesis in America*, London: Routledge.

Saltvedt, S., Almström, H., Kublickas, M., Valentin, L., Bottinga, R., Bui, T.H., Cederholm, M., Conner, P., Dannberg, B., Malcus, P., Marsk, A. and Grunewald, C. (2005) 'Screening for Down syndrome based on maternal age or fetal nuchal translucency: a randomized controlled trial in 39 572 pregnancies', *Ultrasound Obstetric Gynecology*, 25: 537–45.

Sandelowski, M. (1994) 'Channels of desire: fetal ultrasonography in two use-contexts', *Qualitative Health Research*, 4: 262–80.

Santalahti, P. (1996) 'Women's experiences of prenatal serum screening', *Birth*, 23: 101–7.

Scott, S., Prior, L., Wood, F. and Gay, J. (2005) 'Repositioning the patient: the implications of being "at risk"', *Social Science and Medicine*, 60: 1869–79.

Shakespeare, T. (2003) 'Rights, risks and responsibilities', in Williams, S., Birke, L. and Bendelow, G. (eds) *Debating Biology: Sociological Reflections on Health, Medicine and Society*, London: Routledge.

Snijders, R.J., Noble, P., Sebire, N., Souka, A. and Nicolaides, K.H. (1998) 'UK multicentre project on assessment of risk of trisomy 21 by maternal age and fetal nuchal-translucency thickness at 10–14 weeks of gestation', *Lancet*, 352: 343–6.

Statham, H. (1993) 'Serum screening for Down syndrome: some women's experiences', *British Medical Journal*, 307: 174–6.

Statham, H., Green, J.M. and Kafetsios, K. (1997) 'Who worries that something might be wrong with the baby? A prospective study of 1072 pregnant women', *Birth*, 24: 223–33.

Swaan de, A. (1990) *The Management of Normality: Critical Essays in Health and Welfare*, London: Routledge.

Swedish Council on Technology Assessment in Health Care (1998) *Rutinmässig ultraljudsundersökning under graviditet* [Routine ultrasound screening during pregnancy] (SBU-rapport nr 139). Stockholm: SB Offset AB (in Swedish).

Swedish National Board of Health and Welfare (1996) *Hälsovård fore, under och efter graviditeten* [Health care before, during and after pregnancy]. Stockholm: Socialstyrelsen (in Swedish).

Tymstra, T. (1991) 'Prenatal diagnosis, prenatal screening and the rise of the tentative pregnancy', *International Journal of Technological Assessment in Health Care*, 7: 509–16.

Van Teijlingen, E.R., Hundley, V., Rennie, A.M., Graham, W. and Fitzmaurice, A. (2003) 'Maternity satisfaction studies and their limitations: "What is, must still be best"', *Birth*, 30: 75–82.

Williams, C., Alderson, P. and Farsides, B. (2002) 'Dilemmas encountered by health practitioners offering nuchal translucency screening: a qualitative case study', *Prenatal Diagnosis*, 22: 216–20.

Williams, S. (1997) 'Modern medicine and the "uncertain body": from corporeality to hyperreality?', *Social Science and Medicine*, 45: 1041–9.

7 Imaging technology and the detection of 'cold aneurysms'

Illness narratives on the Internet

Gunilla Tegern

Introduction

Medical knowledge and technological innovations are continuously transforming medical practice and our understanding of health, disease, the normal and pathological (Webster 2002). Some of the medical technologies of today, such as the X-ray, seem to be paradoxical in that they can simultaneously be considered as the latest and most sophisticated version of an ongoing development of old and well-established tools and techniques, as well as new innovations that transform medical practice. In order to discover disease at even more early stages, certain diagnostic technologies, for example new imaging methods, tend to move the boundary for what is regarded as normal (Prior 2001). One consequence of this development is that it forces an increasing number of people without symptoms, but diagnosed as being 'at risk', to take decisions to change their life styles or to undergo treatment in order to prevent potential illness in the future.

However, in late modern society we may regard the life of everybody as increasingly influenced by medical knowledge and technological innovations, as suggested by classical studies of the medicalization process (Zola 1983) and more recently observations of enhancement technologies (Elliott 2003). Yet, medical sociologists maintain that we at the same time can observe a decline in medical authority over patients in welfare states and a 'deprofessionalisation' process (Coburn and Willis 2001). Researchers have claimed that the demystification of medical knowledge plays a crucial role in this process. Demystification is supposed to take place when medical knowledge is reproduced in a form that makes it amenable to lay scrutiny (Weiss and Fitzpatrick 1997). In a study in Britain, Weiss and Fitzpatrick observed some consequences of this trend on how GPs experienced their situation and conclude that: 'The greater perceived challenge to clinical autonomy comes, not from proletarianisation in the sense of managerial controls over the content of work but from deprofessionalisation through lay challenges to professional expertise' (1997: 324).

The image of recent shifts in the relationship between medical experts and their patients are however both complex and contradictory. Here, I will confine myself to three trends that may influence medical as well as lay knowledge. First, the patient's view has become a more important issue in health policy (Coulter and Fitzpatrick 2001). In North America as well as in European countries, evidence of failure in medicine to convey information to patients in a satisfactory way has been documented over a long time (ibid.). This may, together with efforts throughout recent decades in several Western countries to reorganize their health care systems towards increased consumerism (Light 2001), have contributed to a change in the representation of the patient. Former representations of the patient as passive, both in health policy discourse and in health research, has gradually lost its hegemonic position to the representation of the patient as actively information seeking and able to take responsibility for his or her own health (Henwood *et al.* 2003).[1] In some countries, a new kind of doctor–patient relationship has been proposed, with implications for the process of informed decision making (Charles *et al.* 2000, Henwood *et al.* 2003). In this informed model, it is assumed that patients are able to 'take decisions that reflect both their preferences and the best scientific knowledge available' (Charles *et al.* 1997: 683). The question of how people could get hold of relevant health information independent of their doctors has thus become a burning question in the health policy discourse in several countries.

Secondly, the general view on knowledge in modern societies is assumed to have undergone a major shift. Theorists, such as Giddens (1990, 1991), argue that modernity is distinguished by a new kind of reflexivity which means that social traditions are continuously contested and revised in the light of new knowledge. This kind of reflexivity includes a new understanding of knowledge which Giddens describes in the following way:

> Doubt, a pervasive feature of modern critical reason, permeates into everyday life as well as philosophical consciousness, and forms a general existential dimension of the contemporary world. Modernity institutionalises the principle of radical doubt and insists that all knowledge takes the form of hypotheses: claims which may very well be true, but which are in principle always open to revision and may have at some point to be abandoned.
>
> (Giddens 1991: 3)

This view on knowledge is echoed in the deprofessionalization debate when 'deprofessionalization is seen as part of a more general social trend in the demystification of expert knowledge' (Weiss and Fitzpatrick 1997).

Third, the emergence of what Castells (2001) describes as a new social form, the network society, implies an increased public access to new technology for knowledge production, distribution and reception. For example, the Internet, a medium of communication that came into general use as late as around 1995, has increased the possibilities to communicate and circulate information incredibly. For the first time in history, Castells points out, it is possible for many persons to communicate to many, at a chosen point of time and on a global scale. The number of people who report that they use the Internet is continuously increasing. In Great Britain, 64 per cent of households in social class one and 48 per cent in social class two reported the ownership of home computers and use of Internet at home at the end of the last century (Hardey 1999). In the year 2000, more than 80 per cent of households in the US reported they used the Internet every week (Castells 2001) and in 2005, 83 per cent of the Swedish population aged 16–75 years reported that they used the Internet. Due to lack of resources as well as poverty and illiteracy it will however be a long time before most people in the world have access to this new medium of communication.

In the health policy discourse in many Western countries, great hopes are set on electronic media such as interactive TV and the Internet. They are regarded as promising means that may solve the problem of patients lacking enough information to be able to make informed decisions about their health.[2] Some researchers stress this view. For example Eysenbach supports a positive view of the role of information technologies, such as the Internet, in the field of health:

> Information technology and consumerism are synergistic forces that promote an 'information age healthcare system' in which consumers can, ideally, use information technology to gain access to information and control their own health care, thereby utilising healthcare resources more efficiently.
>
> (Eysenbach 2000: 1714)

Thus, these three conditions – the change in the view of expert knowledge, seeing people as responsible for their own health and the emergence of new information technologies – will without doubt have consequences for the role of lay as well as medical knowledge and the nature of the information environment. For example, the circulation of medical knowledge, which used to be inaccessible, on the Internet has increased enormously in the last few years. But the Internet is not just a place for official and professionally produced or controlled information. The Internet offers a mixture of health related material, produced for very different reasons and by different agents such as big drug companies, small health firms, lay people, patients, support or activist groups, medical professional authorities, professional pressure groups or governmental authorities. Hardey points out that 'Within it the boundaries around medical science, the health professions and non-orthodox approaches to health are blurred' (2002: 44).

As the Internet offers interactive communication opportunities, information is increasingly circulated in a range of ways, from chat rooms and newsgroups to homepages, mail lists and Internet kiosks. How, then, is it possible for lay persons to navigate in this plethora of health related information? According to Hardey, individuals searching health information on the Internet 'dynamically access the usefulness and quality of the information they collect' (1999: 832). A study by Eysenbach and Köhler (2002) indicates however that we do not remember which websites we retrieve information from. Henwood *et al.* (2003) draws a similar conclusion from a study of mid-life women. Also Hardey has found that we can 'move between web sites that originate in different countries and continents without realising that we have left the site we first accessed' (1999: 826). Rather, we are constructing our own new narrative, a hypertext, when we go along (ibid.: 828).

In the 'informed patient discourse' it sometimes seems as if it is possible for us to avoid the influence of implicit messages in advertisement, the taken for grantedness in dominant discourses or the familiarity of core icons of occurring representations when we are dealing with information and making our choices. The informed patient discourse assumes a careful examination and a weighing of alternatives (Mechanic 1989). Furthermore, a rationally informed choice is sometimes regarded as a choice which is based on relevant 'true' beliefs (Savulescu and Momeyer 1997). Hardey (1999), on the other hand, argues that his research on a group of healthy Internet users supports Giddens' idea that people in late modernity act as self-reflexive consumers who search for information from various sources to make reasonably informed choices. It should be noticed that Hardey talks about a *reasonably*, and not a *rationally*, informed choice. But what kind of behaviour did the participants in his study demonstrate? Were they engaged in strategies to search for the truth (in a philosophical sense)? Or did they primarily weigh pros and cons of the information they had collected? His data rather indicate the latter. They evaluated different standpoints and sometimes even challenged expert knowledge. This discussion on people's strategies as they make choices amounts to that most people in late modernity may be influenced by what Giddens describes as a principle of radical doubt, and they may now and then insist that all knowledge takes the form of hypotheses. This does not necessarily mean that we no longer are involved in maintaining and creating discourses and social representations and are influenced by them in our selection and evaluation of health information and decision-making concerning our health.

Visitors to the Internet can be more or less aware of who stands behind one or another particular standpoint, as Henwood *et al.* (2003) describe in their study of women in mid-life, but yet hardly avoid being influenced by the multitude of different discourses and representations concerning a certain health condition. A specific representation of a condition on the Internet may be a result of a conscious effort by a pressure or activist group in opposition to an official one, as has been shown for example in the case of HIV/AIDS (Gilette 2003). Others may emerge as an unintended consequence of the ways people try to make sense of their illness experiences on the Internet. Both types of representations may influence the decisions of others when they, at a fateful moment due to a serious condition, are searching for more information.

The number of studies that focus on health and the Internet are increasing, but according to Seale most of this research has so far dealt with either 'the relationship of people to health information on the internet, the dynamics of virtual communities in web-hosted discussions and supports groups' or 'the narrowly defined issue of accuracy or quality of information as defined by medical interests' (2005: 516). We still need, Seale argues, more sociologically informed studies of Internet health representations.

Narratives about aneurysms

This chapter draws on a study of illness experiences and representations in illness narratives on the Internet. All the stories deal with a condition in the brain due to a deformation of an arterial vessel, an *intracranial aneurysm* or *brain aneurysm*. In medical science and practice, intracranial arterial aneurysm is today regarded as an acquired lesion in which a possible genetically determined weakness in the vessel wall develops into a ballooning appendage to the vessel (Tegern and Flodmark 2003). An aneurysm may result in sudden death or severe symptoms indicating that the aneurysm is bleeding. Progress in the medical imaging speciality has however resulted in more and more people without any symptoms or signs of disease, completely unexpectedly finding out that they have such a biological abnormality in their brain.

If persons who are suffering from bad headaches due to a diagnosed brain aneurysm want to understand more about their condition as they are waiting for further tests and surgical intervention, they can turn to the Internet. This also goes for those who are waiting to recover after surgical intervention due to a bleeding brain aneurysm or persons without any symptoms who have been told that they have an arterial brain aneurysm after a computer tomography. The search string 'aneurysm AND brain' will result in more than 100,000 hits. Besides strictly scientific homepages about aneurysm and vascular malformation, the patient will find various types of information sites addressing patients and their relatives. One of those is 'Brain Aneurysm Narrative-site', linked to the Aneurysm Support Homepage. In April 2005, more than 800 aneurysm narratives were published on this site, written by people with symptomatic or non-symptomatic intracranial aneurysms, by survivors after a ruptured or bleeding aneurysms, by people with preventively treated aneurysms and by relatives to those who died from it. Every new narrative, the date of publication and the author's name or pseudonym and e-mail address is attached chronologically to a constantly growing list at the rate of approximately two new narratives per week. By clicking on a title the visitor to the site will go to the individual story.

The analysis in this chapter is limited to stories on the Brain Aneurysm Narrative-site. This makes the conditions for the analysis a bit different from some of the earlier studies of illness narratives on the web. Two things usually characterize homepages encompassing illness stories. First, they are only occasionally linked together (Hardey 2002). Those who are looking for such material on the web are forced to spend a lot of time finding sites.[3] Second, many homepages with illness stories do not exist for long, and others are continuously reorganized and old information deleted (ibid.). But this does not characterize the illness narratives on the Aneurysm Support Homepage. The homepage has existed since 1996 and the narratives on the Brain Aneurysm Narrative-site are accessible to everybody in their original form. Furthermore, the site offers easy access to all of the more than 800 narratives which are neatly ordered with a more or less informative heading.

Usually, media studies are classified as a production, representation or reception study (Seale 2003). In studying the Internet, this distinction is sometimes hard to maintain as this new media offers interactive forms of communication. Some places on the Internet offer no more interactive opportunities than a traditional health brochure, and it is easy to distinguish between representations, producers and recipients. But in other cases the three are intertwined.

The Brain Aneurysm Narrative-site is not constructed as a chatroom allowing visitors to take part in current conversation and in that sense interactive. But it is evident from the stories that many storytellers have first visited the site and read the stories before posting their own. It is also evident that the contributors have started to communicate with each other on the 'narrative Internet stage', as well as behind the stage, by sending e-mails to each other. They are in this sense both recipients and producers and, I would argue, co-creators of a representation of aneurysm.

The illness narratives on this site belong to a mixed genre. They are not the result of an interview, but neither are they part of a naturalistic face-to-face conversation. Rather, they are influenced by the diary format, at the same time as they are presented to a selected but unknown audience. This involves, as Hardey points out, 'a blurring of the distinction between the private world of the self manifest in the homepage and the public world of the Internet (2002: 43). All the illness stories are 'molded by rhetorical expectations that the storyteller has been internalizing ever since he first heard some relative describe an illness', as Frank points out (1995: 3) and thus they blur the difference between the public and the private.

Writing and publishing the narratives on the Internet site seems to serve several purposes such as making sense of upsetting experiences, reconstructing identities and sharing experiences with others in a similar situation. In a study of personal homepages that contain accounts of illness, Hardey (2002) distinguishes between four different kinds: (1) narratives which primarily were constructed to explain illness and the consequent emotional and social changes, (2) those which give expert advice to others who have the same or a similar condition, (3) those which promote a particular approach to an illness, or indirectly and finally (4) those that directly sell products through the Internet. On the Brain Aneurysm Narrative-site, the authors in addition to telling their own story also ask for help or give advice to the assumed 'known strangers'. By and large, Frank's (1995) observation that by telling their stories, ill persons offer themselves as a guide to the self-formation of others seems to describe very well what the authors on this site are doing.

When people account for their illness, they articulate their experiences, perceptions and understandings (Hydén 1997). The following analysis of these experiences, perceptions and understandings is guided by two theoretical perspectives – phenomenology and the theory of social representations. I will first describe the technological preconditions for the diagnosis of intracranial aneurysm. Then I will present a more detailed account of the clinical condition concerning a bleeding or rupturing aneurysm, and also an analysis of patients' and relatives' experiences of a bleeding, ruptured or treated aneurysm. Finally, I will deal more closely with some social representations of brain aneurysms that have emerged on the studied Internet site, and discuss how conceptions of the condition as an 'embodied risk' have a potential to intervene in the ambiguous clinical situation and make even patients without symptoms ask for, or comply with, hazardous intervention in order to reconstruct normality.

Intracranial aneurysms and their technological preconditions

On 8 November 1895, the German physicist Wilhelm Conrad Röntgen accidentally discovered some special kind of rays. It turned out that these so-called X-rays were able to make certain kinds of internal structures of objects stand out as shadows against a fluorescent screen or photographic plate. Only a few days after Röntgen had for the first time communicated his discovery in a scientific context, the European and American general public could read about this in the daily press. And in February 1896 an important media event occurred when Thomas Edison tried to X-ray the human brain in front of an assembled press audience (Jülich 2002).

Röntgen's discovery was a condition for the construction of the X-ray apparatus, the birth of an entire new discipline, radiology, and for the creation of a new medical profession with interpretation of images as a speciality (Pasveer 1989). Less than ten years after Röntgen's discovery, a German–Austrian physician published the results of his intensive efforts to apply the X-ray technique on the skull. But it took several decades of discoveries, innovations and experimenting on animals, patients and dead bodies before the technology and its users had the capacity to disclose safe information about the interior of the skull – despite Edison's 1896 efforts in front of the media audience. Not until the technique to inject air or some substances opaque to X-rays 'in the body normally "mute" to X rays' (Fishgold and Bull 2002: 17) was invented, could radiologists start to visualize various pathological abnormalities in the brain on a more regular basis.

In medical practice, doctors knew (through post mortem examination) before the invention of X-ray technology that human beings could present balloon-shaped deformations in a vessel wall, so-called intracranial aneurysms. Autopsy studies have shown that approximately 5 per cent of the general population have or will have intracranial aneurysm (which means about 10–15 million persons in the US or 400,000 in a small country such as Sweden). An aneurysm may start to bleed or rupture, but estimations based on various data suggest that most intracranial aneurysms do not rupture (Wiebers 1998).

As already mentioned, since the 1920s X-ray technology has included techniques for injection of contrast agents into blood vessels. These techniques also make it possible to produce X-ray images of brain vessels by so-called angiography. But it was not until computer technology at the beginning of the 1970s revolutionized medical imaging and gave rise to new imaging methods such as computed tomography (CT), that intracranial aneurysm could be identified and localized with any precision.[4]

Patients' experiences of a dangerous condition

Under certain circumstances (as yet unknown) an arterial aneurysm can rupture and give rise to an arterial haemorrhage into surrounding tissues. If an arterial aneurysm is located on one of the intracranial arteries, a haemorrhage into the brain can be catastrophic with immediate death in about 20 per cent of the cases (Wiebers 1998). For some this may occur without any previous warning and shock their loved ones. In one of the many illness narratives on the studied website written by a relative or friend, a man tells us about his experiences of such an event in the following way:

> My Sister, died on 20 January 1997 at the age of 47 as the result of a sudden cerebral aneurysm. Her death was unexpected and a great shock to all of her family and friends. Except for a severe headache that day no unusual symptoms warned anyone what to expect. Routine for that Sunday was a quiet dinner out with her husband and long time friends. While still at the house she complained of sudden nausea. She suddenly and unexpectedly collapsed. The paramedics were called and arrived within minutes. Rushed to the hospital a short distance away there was nothing that could be done.

Accounts of this kind, about how a healthy person in the middle of her or his life, without any previous warning, is struck by unexpected death, readily catch our attention in everyday life. On closer consideration perhaps most of us will remember how this has happened to somebody known to us: a famous football player, a friend of a friend or perhaps a neighbour. The fact that even a young person without any foreboding may drop down dead will often bring these stories far beyond the close circle of relatives and friends to a wider social world. There, these stories will be added to the collective memory of dramatic events – but not necessarily attached to its medical label aneurysm.

Before the discovery of X-rays, and the constitution of a group of medical specialists able to interpret the shadow images, only a few attempts to intervene surgically had been carried out on the human brain (Fishgold and Bull 2002). However, during the twentieth century neurosurgery has benefited from the developments in radiology and gradually become able to offer surgical treatment for an increasing number of conditions of the brain. Some of those who survive a ruptured aneurysm can, thanks to some acute neurosurgical or endovascular intervention, recover without suffering from any after-effects.[5] But among survivors you often find significant morbidity. Many who due to the haemorrhage lose their ability to move around recover after some time, but often continue to suffer from cognitive problems or problems related to the self. Even if these problems are not always immediately observed by other people, they are very obvious for the suffering person, as this woman writes:

> During the day of May 26th 2003, I was going about my normal daily tasks, of managing two real estate offices, which I owned. I drove from one office to the other, to check on the staff, and was about to leave when one of my staff asked me to look at an email from one of the tenants. I read it and suggested that I could answer if for her. I sat down behind her desk and suddenly was racked with this incredible pain in my head. I passed out, and was revived some 15–20 minutes later by the medical staff in the centre, vomiting and with loss of bladder control ... So unexpected. How my life changed in a split second. ... What would the future bring. I have had to learn to do other things to keep my mind active, sewing and knitting for the new baby. I cannot deal with any form of conflict, and loose concentration. I used to sleep the night through, now I wake sometimes on the hour. I cannot deal with traffic, so am unable to drive. I have no inclination or motivation for the tasks associated with running my own business. I have difficulty remembering simple things like making a favourite recipe. I don't have any feelings of being grateful for getting a second chance at life, something that my specialist confirmed happens to a lot of aneurysm survivors.

This woman, like many other storytellers on the website, describes how the ruptured aneurysm in one second changed her life for ever. After having survived a treated ruptured aneurysm many of the storytellers experience, just like this woman, remaining symptoms or more correctly, after-effects. When the medical philosopher Kay Toombs suggests that 'symptoms of illness are the patient's reports of what is experienced as an alien body sensation' (Toombs 1992: 33), she is referring most of all to experiences such as pain and bodily weakness. But people who are living with a post-ruptured aneurysm are generally referring to other kinds of sensations or experiences. These after-effects are often experienced as a blend of strange feelings and a surprising inability to function, as a female lawyer describes in her narrative:

> As soon as I tried to do any 'real' legal work, researching and in particular, legal writing, I drew a complete blank. I just could not do it. I felt incredibly strange and scary. I did not know what was happening or why, but I just could not write. My brain felt too small, it felt as if I was not at all as smart as I used to be, and I just could not wrap my brain around the issues.

In the case of ruptured aneurysm, the after-effects are thus not experienced as just alien body sensations, but as sensations of an alien self. At the level of immediate experiences, illness manifests itself essentially as a disruption of the lived body (Toombs 1992). The body is no longer behaving in a way the person used to take for granted. Survivors of ruptured aneurysm are not just describing the inability to engage in the world in the ways they are used to, due to pain or stiffness, but also describe that their mind, or brain, is no longer behaving in the way they took for granted that it should. A recurrent element in the stories is how *the self* in a problematic way has come to the forefront and become a more or less permanent thematic object of attention.

It has long been considered that the only possible preventive treatment of a discovered aneurysm located on a brain vessel is to exclude the aneurysm from the vascular system by surgery. But such a treatment concurrently poses the risk of ending up with the same damage that a rupture may cause. In other words, diagnosing and treating a non-ruptured aneurysm may lead to a natural process being successfully intercepted and the patient's life being saved and permanent damage prevented, or it may result in the opposite, i.e. the intervention may trigger the kind of consequences that it should prevent (Wiebers 1998). An example of the latter is described in the narrative of a woman whose aneurysm was accidentally discovered. The doctors offered her surgical intervention and she chose this alternative in order to eliminate the risk that the aneurysm would burst in the future and lead to serious secondary effects:

> My aneurysm was found purely by accident. I had been having migraines since I was 13 years old just after a bad auto accident in which my face was crushed. I went to the doctor in 1991 for the millionth time. The doctor asked when I had had a work-up (I never had). She sent me for CT Scan. There was a big black spot right in the middle of my head … There was an aneurysm. Surgery was scheduled but postponed and scheduled again. … My aneurysm was successfully clipped and I am recovered. Sometimes I don't feel recovered. … It's been 5 years now and I still have bad vision, bad hearing, some involuntary movement in my left fingers, headaches etc. I was a bank teller before and a while after

surgery. I went back to work after 3 months because my doctor said she wanted me to be a productive citizen. I can't think quickly enough and I can't see numbers correctly sometimes so I was out of balance a lot. Finally I either had to quit or get terminated. I chose to quit.

My thought process is slow and my short term memory plays tricks on me. I think I know what I'm doing, but I really don't. I look good, and I act normal so everyone thinks I am normal. I'm far from it, but I can't convince SSDI or even some family members. I'm depressed most of the time and take medication forever.

I wish I could just be me and everyone would understand who I am. Thats what it feels like. Like I am a total stranger in Jetty's body and everyone thinks shes in here. Jetty as I know her is no longer in this head and body. The Jetty I know is a good bank teller and can do anything she wants to. I'm a healthy happy person that everyone goes to for advice. Not this leftover piece of me, without a job and probably will never have one. I feel so helpless.[6]

This woman writes, like many of the others, that the scheduled operation resulted in permanent after-effects of the same kind as those that sufferers from ruptured aneurysms talk about. She hardly agrees with her doctors that the result was successful. She took a risk in order to avoid another. Her narrative supports the interpretation that her expectation of the operation was to reconstruct normality, that is, to become the same person as she was before she had the information about her aneurysm, a person without risk. But instead of experiencing that her biographical normality was reconstructed by the neurosurgical intervention, she is now permanently experiencing lived illness. In many of the narratives this longstanding lived experience of illness is described as a characteristic way of being, a way of being which, with Toombs' words, ' incorporates such characteristics as a loss of wholeness, a loss of certainty, a loss of control, a loss of freedom to act, and a loss of the familiar world' (1992: 90).

Some storytellers describe their experiences as a permanent divorce between their body and their self, or as some of them express it, between self and mind. The woman quoted above expresses a despair that derives from the fact that she still, several years after intervention, seems a stranger to herself, not because her head and body seem to be different but because her proper self was changed with the operation. Intervention in case of a bleeding or rupturing aneurysm may save the patient's life and restore health. But many illness narratives indicate that both preventive intervention and the choice to wait and see may have disastrous consequences for the life of the sufferer. Both choices may end up in chronic illness of a kind similar to traumatic brain injury (TBI). In TBI, as David Webb has pointed out, 'the brain-damaged person cannot readily overcome disability with the assistance of the technological aids available to those whose handicapping condition is physical' (1998: 541). The fact is that these illnesses that primarily affect the mind have a certain significance at a time of a 'mentalist celebration of intellect, the triumph of even an almost disembodied mind over material impediment' (1998: 547).

Living with cold aneurysms

More recently, the available technology has been improved, and the diagnosis can be made much more easily due to development in imaging methods such as CT and magnetic resonance imaging (MRI), which can produce three-dimensional computed information about the brain. The most important feature of these techniques is the enormously increased sensitivity.[7] Today, the sensitivity and specificity of these new imaging methods are in fact so high that small aneurysms can be reliably discovered even before they rupture, so-called 'cold' aneurysms. The ease by which these 'cold' aneurysms are discovered creates new challenges as the natural history, and hence the risk of a fatal bleed, of the condition is largely unknown (Wiebers 1998). Of particular interest is the situation people find themselves in when the improved medical imaging technique not as in the standard situation confirms or disconfirms a suspected aneurysm, but delivers unwarranted information about an aneurysm that nobody suspected or asked for.

For example, if a quite healthy person, without any symptom of a disease, has a bad fall or a bang on the head, X-ray examination is often done to ensure that the knock did not cause bleeding in the brain. In such a situation, the new efficient medical imaging methods can rapidly show that this is not the case, at the same time as they may disclose that the patient has a few millimetres big balloon-shaped deformation on one of the vessels of the brain. And from that very moment, when the 'cold' aneurysm appears on the screen and presents itself to the neuroradiologist, there is somebody who knows. This situation, the visualization of the aneurysm as a result of technological advancement within radiology, unwarrantedly 'forces' itself on the doctors involved, creating problems for both doctors and patients. In Webster's words, medical technology creates patients without symptoms, the 'worried well', who occupy what we might call a therapeutic limbo, adding new forms of ambiguity and risk for both physicians and those subject to their gaze (Webster 2002: 445).

In one of the few published studies on this specific topic, van der Schaaf *et al.* (2002) measured health-related quality of life and psychological state in 21 patients who were aware of having a 'cold' aneurysm or arteriovenous malformation. Compared with the reference population, these patients had a reduced health and quality of life in several dimensions. While standard questionnaires are widely used to obtain subjective assessment of health, and are useful as indicators, they shed no light on the meaning of respondents' answers (Mallinson 2001). In most of the narratives linked to the Aneurysm Support Homepage the authors deal with their experiences of bleeding, rupturing or intervened aneurysms, but there are also some that address the *limbo situation* of having been told about the shadow image of their brain and left to live with the 'boundary uncertainty' of medicine. Most of those who have used the possibility to publish their story on the homepage write about their suffering as well as about their 'decision' to go through an intervention. A young mother diagnosed with a 'cold' aneurysm expresses her view on herself, her life and her health in the following way:

> I am the 31 year old mother of 3 little girls and a wife to my husband Scott. In July I found out that I have a 4 mm wide neck aneurysm in my brain and have had all the tests done since. Angiogram, 2 spinal taps, MRI and a MRA done. Next week the 4th of September I head back to my aneurysm specialist who will decide my fate so to speak.
>
> I have been told that it is unlikely that my aneurysm will rupture, about 1% chance per year, but I've apparently had it for 31 years so doesn't that make it a 31% chance? Anyway, I am worried that my neurologist will tell me to wait and have another MRI in a year ... this has seriously changed my life. The quality of my life is not the same, I run to the ER every time I get a headache, I live in constant fear that it will rupture. I want it taken care of now, I don't want to wait around to see if I'm going to be a statistic or if I end up having to have surgery 30 years from now when my body may not be so healthy.

This woman writes that she has been told that it is unlikely that her aneurysm will rupture. Still she has tried on her own to calculate the risk that this will happen. Without having observed the medical encounter in this specific case, we cannot know what role the woman herself played in the process which ended up with an intervention (according to her updates). But if we consider the fear she expresses we can imagine that she has put a lot of pressure to act on her medical doctors in the clinical encounter. In their study, van der Schaaf *et al.* (2002) found that a number of different indicators of health had changed, suggesting that the lives of the patients had significantly changed, despite the fact that none of them appeared to have lost any abilities. It is possible to argue that the mere knowledge about an aneurysm and the associated risks will transfer the patient into a state of mind that we can call being 'at risk'.

Framing expectations: the social representation of aneurysm as an embodied risk

Social science studies conclude that discourses about risk have become a persistent part of life in modern culture and a dominant way to interpret who gets sick and why (Lupton 1999). Lacking bodily evidence of risk we often perceive our everyday state as a state of no risk (Kavanagh and Broom 1998), but still, everyone is to some extent 'at risk' as Beck (1992) has pointed out.

A distinction between two kinds of health risks is usually made: those arising from the environment and those resulting from individual lifestyle. While environmental risks are regarded as externally imposed on a person, lifestyle risks are related to what a person does or does not do. Anne Kavanagh and Dorothy Broom (1998) have suggested a third kind of risk, embodied risks, or corporeal risks, which they locate in the body of the person who is said to be 'at risk'. This kind of risk imposes a threat from within. While both environmental risks and lifestyle risks just indicate a threatening future disorder, embodied risks signify a disorder simultaneously in the present and the future (1998: 442). And while people may identify themselves as being 'at risk' due to environmental and lifestyle factors, medical technology is a condition for the discovery of an embodied risk and also creates the patient 'at risk'.

As is already evident, a 'cold' aneurysm is not a diagnosis that says something about the causes of signs and symptoms, it is a risk diagnosis. In the clinical encounter the formerly symptom-free individual will be transformed into a patient 'at risk'. Even though we can assume that the doctor in charge will do her best to manage the uncertainty when informing the patient about the condition and prognosis, there is an avalanche of information available in public space telling its own stories. If newly informed patients want to understand more about their condition they can turn to the Internet and find a variety of information sites addressing patients and their relatives. One of these is the already mentioned Aneurysm Support Homepage with the link to the Brain Aneurysm Narrative-site. The homepage has become the cyberspace of a social world. There are many things to say about this social world but here I will confine myself to saying something about conceptions of aneurysm, or to be precise, about some elements in a social representation of aneurysm as an embodied risk that is coming into existence and will potentially influence site visitors that have recently been informed that they have a 'cold' aneurysm.

The social psychologist Serge Moscovici, founder of the theory of social representation, has pointed out that people do not simply perceive and process the information they receive, but also ask questions and seek answers about topics that concern them (Moscovici 1984). According to him and other researchers defending the social representation theory, the cognitivist view of the human being is a simplification because society is not a source of information but of meaning (Moscovici 1984; Joffe 2003). Social representation theory (SRT) offers a way to understand the construction of collective and shared meaning and how common sense and everyday knowledge is produced and structured in public and everyday life. A key concern within SRT is how scientific knowledge about a phenomenon, such as for example 'intracranial arterial aneurysm', will be transformed when it moves from a reified, scientific context to the public space and turns into everyday thinking, a form of knowledge with its own logic. Moscovici (1984, 2000, 2001) has suggested that two fundamental mechanisms influencing this transformation: first what he calls the process of anchoring and second the process of objectification. Moscovici writes:

> Social representations are always complex, and necessarily inscribed within the framework of pre-existing thought ... hence always dependent on systems of belief anchored in values, traditions and images of the world and of existence ... so that every new phenomenon can always be incorporated within explanatory or justificatory models which are familiar and therefore acceptable.
>
> (Moscovici 2000: 156–7)

Without doubt, life and death are the two main themes recurring in all illness narratives on the studied website. Though every illness story is unique and the main themes are individually elaborated, a more or less shared world of meaning may be identified on the site, where both life and death are ascribed a special culturally imprinted meaning. It is not biomedical death that is in the forefront but death as absence and loss of possibilities. This kind of death is not primarily associated with dramatic, historical events and significant public persons, but with everyday man – it is a death that may hit each of us at any time. For those who survive a bleeding aneurysm, death is regarded either as a hardly manageable threat or as a background against which a new life takes shape and sometimes obtains a new value.

Concurrently, death in the emergent representation is given its certain meaning through those who did not survive. Approximately 30 per cent of the narratives are written by the surviving spouse, parents, children and friends. It is by their descriptions of all those everyday routines, reciprocal feelings, common subjects for rejoicing and fears, shared experiences and meaningful memories, future plans etc., that suddenly cease when a person does not survive, that the aneurysm-death obtains a concrete meaning.

But also life obtains a special meaning in this social representation of aneurysm. The 'aneurysm life' falls into three parts: life before the knowledge of aneurysm, life while waiting for something to happen and finally life after a bleeding, a rupture or an intervention. In many narratives significant events, such as a marriage, a completed diploma or a new job, are mentioned and indicate that the storytellers experienced themselves as facing a new promising phase in life when the aneurysm appears. Life before the aneurysm is represented as something rich and promising against which life after gets its meaning.

The second part of the aneurysm life appears as a more or less extended and fateful period while waiting for something to happen, such as a bleeding, an operation, endovascular intervention, or a decision to wait and see. This phase is often described as difficult to put up with and as containing a tension between passive expectations, powerlessness and febrile, dramatic activity. During this period, the biomedical conception of aneurysm is at the centre of attention. In this phase one can expect that the unfamiliar phenomenon in one's head will receive its precise name and localization as an 'aneurysm on the anterior communicating artery' or 'right communicating artery aneurysm'. It will also be visible to oneself on a computer display or an X-ray film. It is also during this phase that the size of the aneurysm in millimetres, and its risk in per cent to rupture and end up in death, will be presented with all the details that one also ought to know. It is now that imaging methods such as angiography, CT and ERC obtain a non-medical meaning that separates the painful examinations from others.

This phase – 'while waiting for something to happen' – appears to be different for those who have had a 'cold' aneurysm discovered by accident and those who have experienced a bleeding or ruptured aneurysm. For the latter group, those who have experienced bodily discomfort, the disease as diagnosed and described by the doctor will however not be identical with the disease they experience themselves. An aneurysm can never be experienced as a change in a vessel wall, even if the patient is able to understand the disease in such a way. The gap that exists between the self and the biomedically defined body has been described excellently by Jean Paul Sartre:

> The problem of the body and its relations with consciousness is often obscured by the fact that while the body is from the start posited as a certain thing having its own laws and capable of being defined from outside, consciousness is then reached by the type of inner intuition which is peculiar to it. Actually if after grasping 'my' consciousness in its absolute interiority and by a series of reflective acts, I then seek to unite it with a certain living object composed of a nervous system, a brain, glands, digestive, respiratory, and circulatory organs whose very matter is capable of being analyzed chemically into atoms of hydrogen, carbon, nitrogen, phosphorus, etc., then I am going to encounter insurmountable difficulties. But all these difficulties stem from the fact that I try to unite my consciousness not with my body but with the body of others. In fact the body which I have just described is not my body such it is for me. [...] So far as the physicians have had any experience with my body, it was with my body in the midst of the world and as it is for others. My body as it is for me does not appear to me in the midst of the world.
>
> (Sartre 1971: 279)

However, when analysing the social representations of aneurysms one can find that new meaning has been added which seems to bridge the gap between the obscure and unfamiliar biomedical conceptions of aneurysm in everyday life and the embodied condition or the lived disease. The storytellers definitely attach great importance to the medical views on aneurysm, all procedures and obscure details. But out of all the many individual stories on the website, a core element in a social representation of aneurysm emerges, where the aneurysm obtains a distinct and significant extra-medical meaning by a kind of marriage between lived experiences and a metaphor.

Those who have had a bleeding or ruptured aneurysm usually describe one or several initial symptoms such as a headache, feeling sick, sensory or visual disturbances. Headache is almost always mentioned, and frequently described as 'the worst headache of my life'. This very common description that is both illustrative and lacking in details is however supplemented by more exhaustive descriptions of experiences of a bleeding or rupturing aneurysm in other illness narratives on the website, as in the following quotation:

> I felt like something was trying to come out of my head, like something was going from the right side of my head to the left and was actually going to come out, there was so much pressure.

This quotation gives us a quite certain image of how it feels when an aneurysm is rupturing. We may on the basis of this description vaguely enter into the feeling that something is trying to come out of our head and presses on the skull from within. The woman's description of the increased pressure can however also be associated with an explosion. Also other storytellers depict their symptoms using an explosion metaphor, as in the two following cases:

> One month ago today, my brain exploded. At least, that is what it felt like ... I felt a slight pressure in my head and then this incredible headache hit me hard. I didn't know what it was, but I knew there was something terribly wrong.

> I bent down to tie my shoe and suddenly there was an explosion in my head. I immediately called 911 for an ambulance, explained to them my condition and shortly after I passed out.

A lot of things may explode: an egg can explode in a microwave oven or a bottle with aerated content can explode in the sun. But the most well-known icon of explosion is a bomb. And quite rightly, you will find authors on the website who go the whole way and use the bomb metaphor when they describe their experiences. One of them expresses herself in the following way:

> All of a sudden it felt that a bomb went off in the back of my head, A truly terrible pain. The worst part was I could not understand what was happening to me, I felt this was far more than my normal migraine. I then passed out in the shower.

The social representation of the ruptured aneurysm as an exploding bomb, which emerges among the narratives, appears to give meaning to the 'cold' aneurysm as well as to the life-threatening unpredictable qualities attributed to this 'silent' condition. As a result the only way to manage this potentially threatening condition seems to be by medical monitoring. A young woman who does not even have a diagnosed 'cold' aneurysm, but whose mother just died of a ruptured aneurysm, thinks about the condition in this way:

> It was a long and difficult process dealing with my mother's death. We now believe that aneurysms run in our family. So far luckily no one else has had one. I now have to deal with the idea that I may have a 'ticking time bomb' in my head. I plan to have the tests run soon, and will go on from there.

In the formation of the social representations on the studied website, the unfamiliar biomedical phenomenon aneurysm has thus been anchored in a well-known cultural icon, the ticking bomb.

Discussion and concluding comments

In this chapter I have presented an analysis of how participants on an illness narrative site on the Internet depict their experiences of ruptured or treated brain aneurysms. I have also explored some core elements in a social representation of the unruptured aneurysm which has emerged on this site. In the context of the production of this social representation, people with experiences of aneurysms become both meaning recipients and meaning producers. Though the stories are written by people who have never met, they influence and are influenced by each other. This can be observed in the way storytellers implicitly or explicitly refer to previous stories and in their updates to subsequent ones. The representation is not emerging out of an individual story but out of the collection of coexisting stories. Albeit the stories elaborate different ideas, they tend to bracket differences and focus on solidarity. Together they reinforce the idea of an aneurysm as a corporeal risk, by mediating a kernel image of a ticking bomb in the brain.

Studies of lay conceptions of cancer have shown that people are using the bomb metaphor also to conceptualize cancer, if the disease is conceived as genetically determined (Robertson 2001, Tegern 1994). In the cancer case however, the bomb metaphor has no direct connection to the nature of the symptoms, nor to the conception of an explosion-like course of events, which sometimes is the case in rupturing aneurysms. In lay conceptions of cancer the metaphor rather stresses the supposedly fixed but hidden time of onset. In the case of aneurysm, the explored kernel image of the representation apparently bridges the gap between the two levels of reality that Sartre (1971) distinguishes as 'the body for others' and 'my body such it is for me'. In the representation, features of the lived disease merge with properties of a well-known cultural icon.[8] For the patient, the representation does not replace given biomedical conceptions and the X-ray visualizations of the condition, or the memory of uneasy sensory sensations that many sufferers from bleeding and rupturing aneurysms experience. The aneurysm, as a condition, becomes loaded with values and emotions of fear and with an imperative to act in favour of medical intervention.

Kavanagh and Broom's (1998) identification of a third type of risk, in addition to lifestyle risks and environmental risks, as something embodied in the individual corresponds with the representation of an aneurysm. Studies of patients being 'at risk' to develop some diseases report that risk has a fundamentally different meaning for the patient as compared with the health practitioners (Kavanagh and Broom 1998, Olin Lauritzen and Sachs 2001). Health risks create a set of challenges for people who are diagnosed, such as translating population characteristics into personal meaning, coping with uncertainty, interpreting the possibility of illness in the non-appearance of symptoms, and mobilizing supervision and risk reduction (Kavanagh and Broom 1998; see also Chapter 6 in this volume). But when we calculate our own health risks we have already taken on board the meaning of risk in our social world, as Joffe (2003) points out.

People construct risks through lenses tinged with elements of group attachment and of experiences of their in-groups and selves, in terms of both the contemporary imagery that they are exposed to and from past misfortunes. These elements do not distort a 'real risk'. Rather, they are the 'reality' in the minds of those who look upon the risks (Joffe 2003: 68). In the case of a 'cold' aneurysm the patient has to calculate and balance two risks, the risk of spontaneous rupture or bleeding and the risk of a rupture or bleeding due to the preventive medical intervention. The symbolic power of the representation works in a direction where every detected small balloon-shaped discrepancy will be considered as disease and risk, as an embodied risk that needs to be eliminated. The image of a ticking bomb submits no place for biding one's time in passivity but promotes different kinds of actions to defuse or eliminate the evil from its place. According to the 'cold aneurysm narratives' the risk of intervention seems to be overshadowed by the risk of rupture and of the unbearable situation of living a life in uncertainty. Surgery seems to be the only way to reconstruct normality.

In search for information, English-speaking patients from all over the world who have been informed that they have a 'cold' aneurysm may enter the 'Brain Aneurysm Narrative-site', pick up ideas and then disseminate elements of the social representation in other public spaces. However, to understand to what extent such a representation really becomes an element in the chain of actions that make up the medical decision process in a concrete case of discovered 'cold' aneurysm, we need a more careful examination of the neuromedical practice. Some tendencies observed in different parts of the Western world support the ideas described here. First, research has shown that aneurysm patients experience a decreased quality of life after just having been informed that they have a 'cold' aneurysm, even if they do not experience any symptoms. Second, patients who have been informed about having a 'cold' aneurysm tend to let the risk of bleeding and rupture overshadow the risk of an intervention. And finally, observations in neuromedical practice indicate that a continuously increasing number of people who are not suffering from any symptoms, are demanding X-ray investigations in order to exclude the possibility that a 'cold' aneurysm is hidden inside their skull.

Acknowledgements

I want to thank Olof Flodmark, Professor in Neuroradiology, who first drew my attention to the problem of cold aneurysm in neuromedical practice and who later invited me to co-operate over the disciplinary boundaries.

Notes

1 For example S. Williams and M. Calnan (1996) have described a similar shift taking place in health research.
2 See for example NHS Direct (2005): 'NHS Direct – Revolutionising access to health information'. Here we can read that: 'NHS Direct is revolutionising the way people access health information and advice... Its strategy "Better information, better choices, better health" is about developing local and national resources to meet everyone's need for health information so as to enable them to make better informed choices about managing their own health and treatment options'. NHS Direct is a 24-hour health advice and information service for England. The NHS Direct website – www.nhsdirect.nhs.uk – attracts more than a million visits each month. In 2004/5 the website attracted nine million visits compared with 1.5 million during its first year in 2000/1.
3 Private homepages may also have problems being ranked among the first in a search. Seale reports that search engines lead people to large sites whose designers have enough knowledge to get their sites ranked among the top 10–20 listed as results (Seale 2005).
4 Godfrey Hounsfield introduced CT in 1971. He was awarded the Nobel Prize for this invention in 1979. Conventional X-ray images are shadow images that cannot reveal the real geometric distribution of organs. A three-dimensional volume will be represented by a two-dimensional projection. 'Computed tomography is a means of obtaining images that portray the real tissue distribution in a single slice. With CT, therefore, a two-dimensional slice is obtained' (Hasman 1997).
5 Recently some neuroradiologists have developed techniques for arterial occlusion with a coil or microballoon. This kind of intervention, which is done from the inside of the vessel and needs no surgery, is only applicable to some cases of aneurysm. Neither of these techniques are without risk.
6 Potential publishers of their narrative on the site are informed in advance that the narratives are added to the list as they are received, without regard to grammar, or literary style. If editing is deemed necessary to ensure accuracy of medical or anatomical terms, it will be implemented with the permission of the author.
7 Computed tomography is about 100 times more sensitive than conventional radiography (Bull 2002: 83). Magnetic resonance imaging (MRI) is based on electromagnetic radiation instead of X-rays. With MRI vessels may be selectively imaged without need of contrast media (Hasman 1997).
8 Moscovici has described the role of metaphors in social representation: 'It appears that metaphors play an important role in the creation of social representations,

precisely because they slot ideas and images which are little familiar into others which are already familiar' (Moscovici 2001: 20).

References

Beck, U. (1992) *Risk Society: Towards a New Modernity*, London: Sage.

Bull, J. (2002) 'The history of computed tomography', in E.A. Cabanis and M.-T. Iba-Zizen (eds) *A History of Neuroradiology*, 3rd edn, Toulouse: Europa Edition.

Castells, M. (2001) *The Internet Galaxy – Reflections on the Internet, Business and Society*, New York: Oxford University Press.

Charles, C., Gafni, A. and Whelan, T. (1997) 'Shared decision-making in the medical encounter: what does it mean? (or, it takes at least two to tango)', *Social Science and Medicine*, 44: 681–92.

Charles, C., Gafni, A. and Whelan, T. (2000) 'How to improve communication between doctors and patients', *British Medical Journal*, 320: 1220–1.

Coburn, D. and Willis, E. (2001) 'The medical profession: knowledge, power, and autonomy', in G.L. Albrecht, R. Fitzpatrick and S.C. Scrimshaw (eds) *Social Studies in Health and Medicine*, London: Sage.

Coulter, A. and Fitzpatrick, R. (2001) 'The patient's perspective regarding appropriate health care', in G.L. Albrecht, R. Fitzpatrick and S.C. Scrimshaw (eds) *Social Studies in Health and Medicine*, London: Sage.

Elliott, C. (2003) *Better Than Well: American Medicine Meets the American Dream*, New York: W. W. Norton.

Eysenbach, G. (2000) 'Recent advances: consumer health informatics', *British Medical Journal*, 320: 1713–6.

Eysenbach, G. and Köhler, C. (2002) 'How do consumers search for and appraise health information on the world wide web? Qualitative study using focus groups, usability tests and in-depth interviews', *British Medical Journal*, 334: 573–7.

Fishgold, H. and Bull, J.W. (2002) 'A short history of neuroradiology', in E.A. Cabanis and M.-T. Iba-Zizen (eds) *A History of Neuroradiology*, 3rd edn, Toulouse: Europa Edition.

Frank, A. (1995) *The Wounded Storyteller: Body, Illness and Ethics*, Chicago, IL: University of Chicago Press.

Giddens, A. (1990) *The Consequences of Modernity*, Cambridge: Polity Press.

Giddens, A. (1991) *Modernity and Self-identity: Self and Society in Late Modern Age*, Cambridge: Polity Press.

Gilette, J. (2003) 'Media activism and Internet use by people with HIV/AIDS', *Sociology of Health and Illness*, 25: 608–24.

Hardey, M. (1999) 'Doctor in the house: the Internet as a source of lay health knowledge and the challenge to expertise', *Sociology of Health and Illness*, 21: 820–35.

Hardey, M. (2002) '"The story of my illness": personal accounts of illness on the Internet', *Health*, 6: 31–46.

Hasman, A. (1997) 'Medical imaging', in J.H. van Bemmel and M.A. Musen (eds) *Handbook of Medical Informatics*, Heidelberg: Springer.

Henwood, F., Wyatt, S., Hart, A. and Smith, J. (2003) '"Ignorance is bliss sometimes": constraints on the emergence of the "informed patient" in the changing landscapes of health information', *Sociology of Health and Illness*, 25: 589–607.

Hydén, L.-C. (1997) 'Illness and narrative', *Sociology of Health and Illness*, 19: 48–69.

Joffe, H. (2003) 'Risk: from perception to social representation', *British Journal of Social Psychology*, 42: 55–73.

Jülich, S. (2002) *Skuggor av sanning: Tidig svensk radiologi och visuell kultur* (Shadows of truth), Linköping Studies in Arts and Science, nr 25, Linköping: Tema Institute (in Swedish).

Kavanagh, A.M. and Broom, D.H. (1998) 'Embodied risk: my body, myself?', *Social Science and Medicine*, 46: 437–44.

Light, D.W. (2001) 'The sociological character of health-care markets', in G.L. Albrecht, R. Fitzpatrick and S.C. Scrimshaw (eds) *Social Studies in Health and Medicine*, London: Sage.

Lupton, D. (1999) *Risk*, London: Routledge.

Mallinson, S. (2001) 'Listening to respondents: a qualitative assessment of the Short-Form 36 Health Status Questionnaire', *Social Science and Medicine*, 54: 11–21.

Mechanic, D. (1989) 'Consumer choice among health insurance options', *Health Affairs*, Spring: 138–48.

Moscovici, S. (1984) 'The phenomenon of social representations', in R.M. Farr and S. Moscovici (eds) *Social Representations*, Cambridge: Cambridge University Press.

Moscovici, S. (2000) *Social Representations: Explorations in Social Psychology*, Cambridge: Polity Press.

Moscovici, S. (2001) 'Why a theory of social representations?', in K. Deaux and G. Philogene (eds) *Representations of the Social*, Oxford: Blackwell.

NHS Direct (2005) 'NHS Direct – Revolutionising access to health information', 29 September. Available at: http://www.nhsdirect.nhs.uk/chq.asp?classid=81&articleID=1219&inthidetitle=1 (accessed 24 January 2006).

Olin Lauritzen, S. and Sachs, L. (2001) 'Normality, risk and the future: implicit communication of threat in health surveillance', *Sociology of Health and Illness*, 23: 497–516.

Pasveer, B (1989) 'Knowledge of shadows: the examination of X-ray images in medicine', *Sociology of Health and Illness*, 11: 360–81.

Prior, L. (2001) 'Review article', *Sociology of Health and Illness*, 23: 251–9.

Robertson, A. (2001) 'Biotechnology, political rationality and discourses on health risk', *Health*, 5: 293–309.

Sartre, J.-P. (1971) *Being and Nothingness: An Essay in Phenomenological Ontology*, 7th edn., New York: Citadell Press.

Savulescu, J. and Momeyer, R.W. (1997) 'Should informed consent be based on rational beliefs?', *Journal of Medical Ethics*, 23: 282–8.

Seale, C. (2003) 'Health and media: an overview', *Sociology of Health and Illness*, 25: 513–31.

Seale, C. (2005) 'New directions for critical Internet health studies: representing cancer experience on the web', *Sociology of Health and Illness*, 27: 515–40.

Tegern, G. (1994) *Frisk och Sjuk. Vardagliga föreställningar om hälsan och dess motsatser* (Everyday conceptions of health and its opposites). Linköping Studies in Arts and Science 119. Linköping, Dep. Health and Society (in Swedish).

Tegern, G. and Flodmark, O. (2003) 'Psychological, social and economical consequences of incidental discovery of aneurysm', *Revista di Neuroradiologia*, 16: 739–42.

Toombs, S.K. (1992) *The Meaning of Illness*, Dordrecht: Kluwer.

Van der Schaaf, I.C., Brilstra, E.H., Rinkel, J.E., Bossuyt, P.M. and van Gijn, J. (2002) 'Quality of life, anxiety, and depression in patients with untreated intracranial aneurysm or arteriovenous malformation', *Stroke*, 33: 440.

Webb, D. (1998) 'A "revenge" on modern times: notes on traumatic brain injury', *Sociology*, 32: 541–55.

Webster, A. (2002) 'Innovative health technologies and the social: redefining health, medicine and the body', *Current Sociology*, 50: 443–57.

Weiss, M. and Fitzpatrick, R. (1997) 'Challenges to medicine: the case of prescribing', *Sociology of Health and Illness*, 19: 297–327.

Wiebers, D.O. (1998) 'Unruptured intracranial aneurysms – risk of rupture and risks of surgical intervention', *New England Journal of Medicine*, 339: 1725–33.

Williams, S.J. and Calnan, M. (1996) 'Modern medicine and the lay populace: theoretical perspectives and methodological issues', in S.J. Williams and M. Calnan (eds) *Modern Medicine: Lay Perspectives and Experiences*, London: UCL Press.

Zola, I.K. (1983) *Socio-Medical Inquiries: Recollections, Reflections, and Reconsiderations*, Philadelphia, PA: Temple University Press.

8   Phenomenology listens to Prozac

Analyzing the SSRI revolution

Fredrik Svenaeus

Introduction

The prescription of antidepressive pharmaceutics has increased rapidly in Western countries during the 1990s. In Sweden, for example, the rate has increased by 600 per cent. In 2004 the prevalence was about 6 per cent, which means that more than half a million Swedes (out of a total population of nine million) were on antidepressive medication.[1]

Given the incidence of depression and other mental disorders, which are indications of recommended pharmaceutical treatment, it is estimated that at least 20 per cent of the Swedish population will be prescribed an antidepressant at some time in their life.[2]

This is quite an astonishing development, which has given rise to much debate, and it calls for different kinds of empirical and conceptual investigations. How are we to understand this dramatic increase? What are the causes and reasons behind it? Are we medicalizing painful experiences and conditions of everyday life? Or have we rather become more able in detecting and treating diseases of the brain?

In this chapter I will aim at providing a phenomenology of the feelings characteristic of depression and anxiety disorders, addressing not the biological underpinnings, but the lived experience and meaning-structures inherent in these feelings. If one wants to understand how anxiety, boredom and grief can develop into pathologies, one needs to address the role they play in everyday human life and culture as *constitutive* phenomena. It is highly unlikely that we will be able to understand the differences between normal and pathological feelings, solely by studying brain chemistry, even though we might become even more able in changing the biology of our brains in a way that make us feel and live better. Psychiatry needs a phenomenological approach to supplement and guide psychopharmacology, as well as to understand its own place and function in contemporary culture and society. This phenomenological approach should in addition to broadening the focus of the psychiatric gaze, also make possible a critical stance towards its methods and goals (Crossley 2003).

SSRIs

One obvious factor behind the increase in question is the introduction of new sorts of antidepressive drugs on the market, which have been prescribed more readily by physicians than the old ones, possibly because of better efficacy, definitely because of less disturbing side effects. These drugs are marketed and promoted quite intensively by pharmaceutical companies, and the information campaigns, targeted at doctors, have been shown to have a quite significant effect on the prescription rate of individuals.[3]

Antidepressants can be divided into different subgroups. The two subgroups of antidepressive drugs which were used before 1990 in Sweden, were the MAOIs (monoamine oxidase inhibitors) and the tricyclics (named after the central three-ring structure of the molecule).[4] These drugs often showed good effects on depression, but they had severe side effects, such as food restrictions, dry mouth, sweating, nausea, dizziness, constipation and sleeping problems.[5] In the 1990s (end of the 1980s in the USA) a new type of antidepressants was introduced – the SSRIs (selective serotonin reuptake inhibitors) – which were made famous by the brand name of Prozac (the chemical name of Prozac is fluoxetine). Fluoxetine was not introduced in Sweden until 1995 (as Fontex), but another SSRI, citalopram (Cipramil, Celexa), was introduced in 1992, and soon gained popularity among doctors and patients in a way similar to what happened to Prozac a couple of years earlier in other countries. Other widely prescribed SSRIs in Sweden are paroxetin (Seroxat, Paxil) and sertralin (Zoloft). Another type of similar antidepressants, affecting the reuptake not only of serotonin but also of noradrenaline in the synapse, is the SNSRIs (selective noradrenaline and serotonin reuptake inhibitors). The most prescribed SNSRI in Sweden, venlafaxin (Efexor), was introduced on the market in 1995, and it has gained steadily in sales since then. Nevertheless, SSRIs account for more than 75 per cent of the prescriptions of antidepressants in Sweden today and the situation appears to be similar in most other countries.[6]

Phenomenology

So how should we understand this – as we might truly call it – SSRI revolution? How should we listen to Prozac?[7] In this chapter I will try to show how phenomenology – the philosophy and research tradition inaugurated by Edmund Husserl roughly 100 years ago – can pave the way for a better understanding of the issues involved in both the development in question and the pro–contra debates surrounding it. By way of introduction, phenomenology might be described as the attempt to found a conceptual apparatus that, in contrast to the disembodied theories and investigations of natural science, is based on lived experience (Spiegelberg 1982, Zahavi 2003). The starting point is everyday life, viewed and investigated from a certain perspective: the phenomenological attitude. What is focused upon in this attitude is often called the *meaning* of experience. Lived experience, on the one hand, and the theories and results of natural science, on the other, are meaningful in entirely different ways; suffering from the ravages of an illness, for example, is something altogether different from coldly cataloguing the characteristics of a disease.[8] Science, as a human activity that strives to solve puzzles and produce new results, is no doubt meaningful, but the manner of explanation particular to science, with its focus on causal relations within nature, is not directly tied to the everyday world. The meaning that phenomenology investigates is not found within the causal patterns of the world studied by science (the brain in the case of SSRIs), but in the subjective perspective the person develops on herself and the world around her in everyday life.

Phenomenology, which started out as a philosophical tradition – the most famous names are Edmund Husserl, Martin Heidegger, Maurice Merleau-Ponty, Jean-Paul Sartre, Paul Ricoeur and Hans-Georg Gadamer – found quick response in other disciplines, such as aesthetics, psychology, sociology, ethnography and pedagogy, and developed into a vast field of different research programs. In the last three decades, phenomenology has also gained some attention within the discipline of medicine (Toombs 2001), and particularly so within psychiatry (Spitzer *et al.* 1993). My phenomenological approach in this chapter should be understood as a conceptual, philosophical analysis, rather than as a piece of qualitative, empirical research, but the analysis is nevertheless linked to interviews with doctors and patients about SSRIs, and to different findings in empirical disciplines about depression and medication.[9]

What should we expect from a phenomenological analysis of the SSRI revolution? Which questions does the analysis need to address to make us better understand the issues involved? One pressing question is the one concerning *normality*. When an SSRI is prescribed this seems to indicate that the patient is suffering from an illness. How is the border between health and ill-health to be drawn regarding the kind of suffering associated with SSRI medication? The phenomenologist addresses this question on the life-world level (illness), and not on the level of biological functioning of the brain (disease). That this approach is particularly fitting in the case of SSRIs, even though the drugs in question, of course, have a biological impact on the serotonin level in the brain, becomes clear when we turn to the models of psychiatric diagnosis. There are no diagnostic tests for serotonin levels in the brain (so far) to be used on patients; instead, doctors rely on clinical experience and diagnostic manuals in their judgments on treatment.[10]

The psychiatric diagnosis

A brief look into one of the two psychiatric bibles for diagnosis, DSM-IV (2000) (the other one is ICD-10 [2004]), reveals what kind of questions and observations are supposed to be made by the doctor in order to decide if the person is suffering from a diagnosis possibly meriting medication.[11] The major diagnostic groups in DSM-IV which are associated with SSRI treatment are depressive disorders, including dysthymia, which is a kind of chronic depressive mood and personality type; and anxiety disorders of different sorts, such as social phobia and post-traumatic stress disorder.

The corner stone of depressive disorders is the presence of what is called "a major depressive episode" (DSM-IV 2000: 356). This means that a depressed mood (sadness, emptiness) and a loss of interest or pleasure have been present most of the day, nearly every day, for at least two weeks, and, in addition to this, that at least three out of seven criteria are also fulfilled for this period. The seven criteria are: significant weight change, insomnia or hypersomnia, psychomotor agitation or retardation, fatigue or loss of energy, feelings of worthlessness or excessive or inappropriate guilt, diminished ability to think or concentrate, and recurrent thoughts of death.

The symptoms in question must also cause "clinically significant distress or impairment in social, occupational, or other important areas of functioning", and they should not be immediately caused by medication or bereavement (loss of a loved one).

If we turn to the anxiety disorders in DSM-IV, we find a corresponding pattern of deviant feelings, problems in world engagement and altered embodiment. The key role here, in the type of disorders treated with SSRIs, is played by panic attacks, which are triggered by being in different alarming situations. A panic attack is specified in the following manner: "a discrete period of intense fear or discomfort, in which four (or more) of the following symptoms developed abruptly and reached a peak within 10 minutes": (1) palpations, pounding heart, or accelerated heart rate; (2) sweating; (3) trembling or shaking; (4) sensations of shortness of breath or smothering; (5) feeling of choking; (6) chest pain or discomfort; (7) nausea or abdominal distress; (8) feeling dizzy, unsteady, lightheaded, or faint; (9) derealization or depersonalization; (10) fear of losing control or going crazy; (11) fear of dying; (12) paresthesias; (13) chills or hot flushes (DSM-IV 2000: 432). The anxiety attacks are recurrent and often associated with being in a special type of situation (meeting and speaking to strangers in the case of social phobia, for instance). The person in question not only experiences anxiety in having the dramatic attacks, but is often also constantly *anxious about* having them.

Although most physicians do not follow these lists of criteria strictly in making their diagnoses, the criteria clearly indicate what kind of matters they investigate in their encounters with patients. Diagnosis, in these cases, is all about phenomenological life-world issues, although the criteria are not developed in any theoretically reflected manner. One of the main points of the development of DSM was, indeed, to make diagnosis without theory (psychoanalytic or biological) possible, so the fact that concepts are not defined or linked to each other in a theoretical manner of explaining the disorders should come as no surprise. This, however, does not mean that we could not proliferate from trying to explain, and especially understand, what kind of mélange a depression or an anxiety disorder is, and what it is that distinguishes them from normal conditions of life. Phenomenology could help us in this task, by offering a kind of understanding that is not preconditioned by scientific models of the psyche, neither of psychoanalytic nor of biological heritage. In the phenomenological attitude, we abstain from theoretical prejudgments and study the way phenomena appear from the first-person perspective. We study their structure of meaning, not the causes behind them.

Which kind of phenomena we should concentrate upon in the case of depression and anxiety disorders is pretty clear from the lists of criteria given in DSM-IV – the central roles in the diagnostic patterns are played by painful feelings, problems with engagement in the world, and altered embodiment. If we could find a way of understanding how these three types of phenomena are related to each other in everyday life, we would have gained much in our attempts to analyze the SSRI revolution. If we, by the same phenomenological analysis, could offer a way to understand the difference between normal and abnormal (meaning healthy and ill) ways of being attuned, world-engaged and embodied, we would have come even further. And if we, finally, by way of the analysis, were able to offer a more extended account of the relation between the *normal* and the *normative* in the sphere of feelings, world-engagement and embodiment – including social processes, patterns of self formation and matters pertaining to the good life – we would certainly gain a rather comprehensive, if not complete, understanding of the SSRI revolution. I will not be able to carry out all these three missions in this chapter, but I will try to make a good start.

Being attuned and being-in-the-world

The three basic feelings which are characteristic of anxiety disorders and depression are, I would say, *anxiety*, *boredom* and *grief*. It is clear from the lists of criteria in DSM-IV stated above that one could certainly choose to give these feelings slightly different names and thereby slightly different meanings. In the case of grief, we could choose to speak about sorrow, sadness, guilt, or loss, for instance. I will try to handle this dilemma in my attempts to draw a line between normal grief and depression below. In specifying the differences between normal anxiousness and boredom, on the one hand, and the pathological forms of these phenomena, on the other, a similar discussion will occur.

It might seem from the diagnostic patterns dealt with above that anxiety disorders and depressive disorders are rather different. One should not forget, however, that anxiousness and panic attacks are common features of depression, and that people who suffer from anxiety disorders often are depressed as well. The fact that SSRIs appear to have good effects on both kinds of disorders could be taken to indicate that the disorders are best understood in a biological manner as failing functions of serotonin reuptake. But a biological approach does not exclude a phenomenological model of understanding. It should be stressed that even if we did know that lack of serotonin is the cause of depression and anxiety disorders in a way similar to the lack of insulin being responsible for diabetes (most neurobiologists and psychiatrists would not support such a conclusion today), this model of understanding would not make a phenomenological approach irrelevant. To know the cause of a phenomenon is one thing, to understand its meaning and phenomenal structure is something different.

One promising place to start looking for a phenomenology of feelings is the philosophy of Martin Heidegger. In his first major work *Being and Time*, originally published in 1927 (1986), and in the lecture course *The Fundamental Concepts of Metaphysics*, given in 1929–30 (1983), Heidegger offers extensive and in-depth analysis of the feelings of anxiety and boredom, respectively. In the two books the two phenomena – anxiety and boredom – are assigned central, and in many way parallel, places and functions. In later works Heidegger also pays deep attention to grief (Haar 1992), and I will return to this aspect of depression below. In what way can we benefit from Heidegger's phenomenological analyses in this context?[12]

The first point I would like to bring forward is the way in which Heidegger makes lucid that certain feelings – moods – are world-constitutive phenomena. Moods open up a world to human beings in which things *matter* to them in different ways. It is common in the contemporary philosophy of feelings to distinguish between sensations, emotions and moods. Sensations have a distinct place in the body (pain, tickling), emotions have an object and are based upon beliefs (love, hate), whereas moods do not have a place in the body and also lack a distinct object, they rather color the way everything appears to the subject (anxiety, boredom and sadness, or joy, curiosity and awe). This schematization has its roots in Aristotle and has been further developed in slightly different ways in the tradition of analytical philosophy (Solomon 1993). What is central to the distinctions is that feelings in the form of emotions get a cognitive content; that is, feelings are not merely passions, which lead the rational agent astray in his search for knowledge, feelings are indeed forms of knowledge in themselves.

Note, however, that this merely holds for emotions – in which an object of the feeling is involved – when it comes to sensations and moods the cognitive content is much harder to pin-point and therefore tends to fall out of the analysis. This might appear rather adequate in the case of sensations, in which the possible cognitive content is so crude in contrast to the content of emotions – for example that my finger hurts in contrast to the emotion of envy towards a certain person, which includes quite elaborate beliefs about the state of the world and the way I would like it to be. When it comes to moods, however, the lack of a distinct object of the mood seems to have forced the classic analysis in the wrong direction. Moods, for sure, do not contain thoughts in the same way that emotions might do, but they nevertheless determine which kinds of thoughts I will be able to develop. Moods are not added on top of thoughts, which I have already formed and which will thus make the thoughts seem happy or sad because I am tuned in different ways. The moods I live in underlie my thought formation rather than being added on top of it; joyfulness and sadness will lead to development of very different kinds of thoughts with different content. This is of course the reason why thoughts of death, guilt and hopelessness typically occur in the life of a depressed person.

To understand the constitutive role of moods more thoroughly we will introduce some basic notions from Heidegger's phenomenology such as they are developed in *Being and Time* and *The Fundamental Concepts of Metaphysics*, notably the concept of being-in-the-world (*in-der-Welt-sein*). The world, for Heidegger, is not a collection of objects in the midst of which we human beings are placed in the same way as a table is placed in a room, which is placed in a building, which is placed in the city of Stockholm, etc. The world is not basically a geographical phenomenon. Nor is it a physical phenomenon, in the sense that we would come to know the most basic structure of the world through doing quantum mechanics or something similar. The world is not the *res extensa* in contrast to the *res cogitans* of the subject. The Descartian, dualistic split is where things started to go wrong in the understanding of the world phenomenon, according to Heidegger (1986: 89ff.).

Instead the phenomenological world concept is to be understood as a web of meaning where every object (or tool as Heidegger calls it) has its place and appears for a human being on the basis of its significance for doing different things. I intend the word "doing" to have a very wide application here; the Heideggerian concept is rather understanding (*Verstehen*). You can do things with words and thoughts, just as you can do things with your hands. The important thing is that in all these cases you handle different things to bring about something, on your own or – most often – with other people. Thus to understand what a hammer is, to use the most well-known example from *Being and Time*, is, on the everyday level, to be able to use it in building something, and, on the phenomenologically reflected level, to see how it relates to other phenomena in the world (nails, boards), from which it attains its special place in a web of meaning (1986: 69ff.). Humans in their being-in-the-world are thus standing in a meaningful relation to the things they are approaching, they are *with* the things and not just beside them and in this being-with-the-things they also assign them meaning in different ways by doing things.

Feelings, especially in the form of moods, in Heidegger's phenomenology, are basic to our being-in-the-world, since they open up the world as meaning-ful, as having significance. They are the basic strata of what Heidegger refers to as *facticity*, our being thrown into the world prior to having made any thoughts or choices about it. We find ourselves *there*, always busy with different things that matter to us, together with other people, and this "mattering to" rests on an attunement, a mood-quality which the being-in-the-world always has (1986: 134ff., 1983: 99ff.). Every activity is attuned in a way that brings out its significance. Meaningfulness in all forms thus has a tune to it. The different moods in question need not be powerful or directly paid attention to, but they are *there* as the constitutive ground of our being placed in the meaning pattern of the world. We do indeed not choose our moods; they come to us and cannot easily be changed.

Anxiety and boredom

Let us now come back to anxiety and boredom. These are quite peculiar moods (or *Stimmungen* as the German language has it). It is striking, and for sure no coincidence, that these two major pathologies of our contemporary life are the very ones to which Heidegger gives the name *Grundstimmungen* in his phenomenological analysis from the late 1920s (Held 1993). What is peculiar to anxiety and boredom is that they not only open, but also *block* our possibilities to be in the world in the manner of being with things and other human beings in a way that makes sense to us. They do this in different ways though. Anxiety has a paralyzing quality to it, whereas boredom rather puts us to sleep. In anxiety the world bursts, in boredom it withers. To Heidegger these disturbing experiences carry important possibilities for phenomenological analysis itself. In anxiety and boredom it becomes possible to catch sight of the very *structure* of the world in its meaningfulness, since it is, so to say, laid bare, as a pure meaning structure in which we can no longer engage. No particular thing in the world matters any more and thus it becomes possible, and even necessary, to address the meaning of the being-in-the-world *as such*. This is the possibility of an *authentic*, philosophically reflected life in Heidegger, which in contrast to the public anonymity of the "they" (*das Man*) faces its own finitude and accepts responsibility for its own choices (1986: 260ff.).

I will return briefly to Heidegger's analysis of authenticity and inauthenticity below. His rendering of the relationship between these two different kinds of understandings, i.e. forms of life, is very complex and insightful, but it nevertheless, I think, suffers from various phenomenological errors, which mainly have to do with Heidegger's treatment of intersubjectivity (Nancy 2003). For the moment, I would like to focus upon two aspects of Heidegger's anxiety- and boredom-analysis, which I think are fruitful for a phenomenology of psychiatry: being at home and being in time. Anxiety, in *Being and Time*, and boredom, in *The Fundamental Concepts of Metaphysics*, are both characterized as *unhomelike* phenomena (1986: 189, 1983: 120). They make the settling, the being at home in the world, impossible, since the world resists meaningfulness. The world becomes alien; it is not *my* world anymore. Heidegger even talks about an eternal home longing (*Sehnsucht*), which is let loose in boredom. The key idea of authentic understanding is to develop this unhomelikeness and home longing to a kind of structural crescendo, from which it is possible to make it productive for philosophical purposes. The problem from the point of view of psychiatry, however, is that one might get stuck in anxiety or boredom as destructive, rather than productive, life experiences. These moods can be so overwhelming that it becomes impossible to return to homelikeness again. Unhomelikeness is a necessary ingredient of life that can be rewarding in many ways, when it makes us see things in novel and more nuanced ways, but it needs to be balanced by homelikeness, if we should not fall into a bottomless pit of darkness (Svenaeus 2001: 90ff.).

Time is a key issue here; single or shorter periods of anxiety or boredom might provide life with greater depth and indeed authenticity, whereas recurrent anxiety attacks and deep boredom, which refuses to go away, transform life in an unhomelike way, which appears to be pathological. It is important to realize, however, that such a focus on time, counting the hours, days, weeks, months, or even years of anxiety and boredom, is not yet a phenomenologically developed understanding of time, such as we find in Heidegger. Phenomenological time is *lived* time, time as our way of approaching the future from out of the past in the meaning-centered now. As the person suffering from anxiety or boredom will know, one second can pass in the blink of an eye, or last for something which feels like an eternity. The latter is, indeed, the case in both anxiety and boredom, although in different ways. In anxiety the now is intensified and concentrated in a way that threatens to implode, whereas in boredom it is infinitely stretched out and inert. In both cases the now resists to let go of the person and forces her back on herself: the now blocks the flow of life, the taking part in, engaging in, the world together with other people. Anxiety and boredom have a lonesome character to them and this is no doubt what fascinated Heidegger, as it has fascinated philosophers since the time of the Greeks. But this non-chosen lonesomeness, which is the result of an attunement that blocks engagement in a world shared with others, is not only a philosophical ideal, it might also develop into something pathological.[13]

Normality: body and world

To approach and try to understand anxiety and boredom from a phenomenological point of view consequently means to focus upon everyday life as a being-in-the-world in which moods play a constitutive role. Being-in-the-world is also a being in time, or rather a being *as* time, in which time is understood in the manner of our engaging in different projects in the world together with other persons. Every thing has its time, since it is a part of the world where we do things. The characteristic aspect of anxiety and boredom, however, is that things no longer find their proper time, since they do not engage us anymore. We become locked into ourselves in an everlasting meaningless, unhomelike now, instead of approaching the future as a source of possibilities related to our past.

Since the world is always a "world with others" (*Mitwelt*) (1986: 118), the pathological forms of anxiety and boredom (as well as the authentic forms in Heidegger's interpretation) are characterized by loneliness. The others, along with the world, become foreign and strange in anxiety and boredom, they do not move and touch us anymore. If some fellow human being still engages me, if I still feel some urge to meet the address of the world in engaging in different projects, I am not totally locked in, and thus I am still somewhat at home. This is not to say that all forms of shared activities would be pleasant or joyful, it is just to underline that the basic problem with anxiety and boredom is that they tend to block our possibilities of being with others, since they fail to connect us to spheres of shared meaningfulness. And there is indeed no private world to be in without the others. All things around us in the world point towards shared practices and projects. You could choose to live as a hermit, but you could not choose to live in your own world (or if you do, you would, indeed, go psychotic).

Moods make what Heidegger calls *transcendence* (stepping out, being in, taking part) to the world of others possible, by opening up a horizon of meaningfulness to live in. Consequently moods are not qualities of a subject in contrast to the qualities of objects belonging to the world surrounding the subject, but rather phenomena which *connect* the subject to the world, making a being-*in*-the-world possible. I have stressed that moods are not chosen freely, but rather come to us as a basic predicament of existence and transcendence. This being the case, however, we seem to be presented with a basic problem in characterizing depression and anxiety as *mood disorders*, as pathologic phenomena, in contrast to the boredom and anxieties of everyday life. If moods are not qualities which essentially belong to the subject – to the self, i.e. person – but rather a structure of transcendence, a way of being-in-the-world, how are we to understand the essential difference between bored and depressed people and between anxious and "overanxious" (that is, disordered, abnormal, unhealthy) people? Why do some people "get stuck" in boredom and anxiety in a way that transforms their being-in-the-world into a pathologic condition of overwhelming unhomelikeness and "locked-inness", whereas others pass through the experiences of boredom and anxiety and are yet able to maintain a homelike being-in-the-world?

I would like to start answering this question by making use of some concepts and distinctions developed by Thomas Fuchs in his study *Psychopathologie von Leib und Raum* (2000). Fuchs introduces the notion of *leibliche Resonanz* – bodily resonance – in explaining how the body "picks up" moods in its transcendence to the world of human projects. The lived body is the central vehicle of our transcendence to the world as a kinesthetic scheme of intentionality, which underlies our doings and understandings on higher cognitive levels (Merleau-Ponty 1945), but it is so by its capability of being affected by the world in getting tuned. The lived body opens up a "mood-space" – a *Stimmungsraum* – in which our being-in-the-world can envelop, and it does so by acting as a kind of physical resonance box for moods, which are so to say still "free floating": that is, which have not yet taken hold of the subject. Fuchs views depression as a *loss* of bodily resonance (2000: 104), which makes the person no longer responsive to the call of the world and thus leads to a failure of transcendence, a being locked in. The lived body is *korporifiziert* in depression, it is alienated as a stiffened, heavy thing, which no longer vibrates and opens up the mood-space necessary for a full-fledged, homelike being-in-the-world.

The obvious associations to music, which are present in Heidegger's discussions of moods, and which are further strengthened by Fuchs's notion of bodily resonance, should not only be taken metaphorically, I believe, but rather as a reference to the most adequate vocabulary available in developing a phenomenology of moods. The closest we might come to describing what it means to be attuned is captured in the experience of how a piece of music sucks us into a pervasive mood, which colors our entire being-in-the-world. This is not to say that vision, smell and sense are not part of the experience of becoming and being mooded, the attunement of human being-in-the-world rests on a bodily scheme in which the separate sense modalities have not yet been singled out, but work together in a primal unity. Continuing Fuchs's analysis I would like to suggest that the lived body could become not only *devoid* of resonance, but also differently tuned in the sense of being more or less *sensitive* to different moods. In cases of anxiety disorders and depression one might describe this condition as a being out of tune, or a being tuned in minor, in the sense of only picking up the anxious, boring and sad tune qualities of the world. This would allow us to elaborate on a spectrum, stretching from a normal resonance of the lived body (the body being able to pick up a wide spectra of different moods), continuing over different kinds of sensitivities, preferences and idiosyncrasies, which might favor certain moods over others (the melancholic or joyful person), to the cases which we would label pathologies, since the body is severely out of tune, or devoid of tune as a tool of resonance.

Grief and guilt

The phenomenological rendering of the lived body as a tool of resonance, indeed, is not only compatible with, but also seems to support, the view that systematic alterations of the physiological organism (as the blocking of serotonin reuptake) could change the attunement of the person and thus also her being-in-the-world. The alien quality of depressed and anxious embodiment fits well with the idea of a disease process conquering the healthy organism. But the homelikeness or unhomelikeness of our being-in-the-world is certainly not only dependent upon what happens in our bodies – it is also dependent upon what happens in the world around us. Anxiety attacks and periods of depression are often triggered by specific events in the world, which may or may not have something to do with the person's biography. Two of the main characteristics of depression are the feelings of grief and guilt. The depressed person seems to suffer the loss of somebody or something, and she often blames herself for this very loss and the feeling of worthlessness it has left behind. Grief could be taken to be a mood (sadness), but in the sense that it is coupled to the loss of an object (or subject) as a form of mourning, it is rather an emotion. It seems, however, that most depressed persons do not know what or whom they are missing and mourning. The grief rather takes on a mood-quality in the sense of coloring and determining the whole being-*in*-the-world of the person in an unhomelike way.

In his famous essay *Mourning and Melancholia*, written in 1915 (1957a), Sigmund Freud is looking for an explanation of the mourning and feeling of self-guilt in depression.[14] His hypothesis is that the reason the melancholic (depressed) person does not know what she is mourning is that the object of the feeling has been repressed and consequently made unconscious. The melancholic has experienced early abandonment by the mother, but this loss was too hard to bear and must therefore be repressed. The feelings of loss, desperation and anger have instead been directed towards the melancholic herself, which explains the feelings of guilt and worthlessness.

Freud is careful in the essay to point out that this is a hypothesis, which is in need of empirical corroboration. It is doubtful that psychoanalysts have been successful in proving Freud to be right on this point, although it remains beyond doubt today that a miserable childhood, involving different kinds of abandonment and abuse, is correlated to a higher risk of developing depression and other forms of mental disorders. But it is also questionable whether such a hypothesis could *ever* be proven by empirical investigations. How would one go about proving the presence of a specific *unconscious* object or thought (my mother, i.e. I blame my mother) behind the feelings of grief and self-guilt? And why would it have to be the mother? Could not later losses in life provoke the same kind of repression if they were severe enough?[15]

The phenomenological field of investigation is consciousness. This field should certainly be expanded to cover the regions of the unconscious that Freud calls the preconscious – that is, the spheres of experience that are not in the center of focal awareness, but rather supports this awareness and which could be *made* conscious by reflection (attunement, embodiment, and the horizonal patterns of meaning constituting the world) (Zahavi 1999: 203ff.). But Freud's main point is, of course, that the repressed domains of our inner life are inaccessible to such a phenomenological reflection. The unconscious represents a system of thoughts, which is inaccessible to consciousness and which is governed by a totally different kind of logic, but which, nevertheless, influences the fashion of our conscious thoughts, feelings and behavior in a forceful way. From a phenomenological point of view, Freud's theory of the unconscious represents hypotheses that are not accessible to investigation, since they can only be approached indirectly by symptoms that do not reveal their origin by themselves. Freud's meta-psychology is similar to natural science in trying to find *causal* explanations for certain phenomena, whereas phenomenologists do not attempt to go beyond phenomena in their investigations. Nevertheless, the presence of grief and guilt in depression is a phenomenal characteristic, which needs to be taken into account in the phenomenological analysis. There is something peculiar about the objectless grief and the senseless self-blame and guilt, which make the depressive mood and being-in-the-world different from the sadness and self-criticism of everyday life.

One way to tackle this issue is to stress that the difference between normal and abnormal anxiety and boredom in the phenomenological model offered above, seems to point in the direction of grief and loss by itself. I have stressed the unhomelike quality of abnormal (pathological) anxiety and boredom, and this unhomelikeness (rooted in an embodiment which is out of tune) is, indeed, grounded in a sort of primary loss. A loss of the world, but also a loss of oneself, since one's identity and life can only be established and carried on in the patterns of being-*in*-the-world. This would also explain why the grief and guilt of depression (and to some extent of anxiety disorders) fail to find "normal" objects (that is, objects and subjects in the world) and instead are sucked inwards towards oneself. The grief of depression is a mood rather than an emotion, since it colors the poor, lonesome world of the melancholic person in its entirety, and in this poorness and loneliness tends to reflect back on the person herself.

Talking about Prozac

Through the phenomenological analysis of anxiety, boredom and grief we have found a way to understand why feelings such as these are, indeed, constitutive of our being-in-the-world, but, nevertheless, can develop into pathologies, in which the subject can no longer engage in a normal being-in-the-world and is confined to a painful unhomelikeness, which will not let go. The borderline between normal and abnormal being-in-the-world can certainly not be drawn in the same way that one measures and determines a too high blood pressure, or detects the presence of a cancer in the body (disease investigations), but this should come as no surprise, given the nature of phenomenological investigations, and the characteristics of mental illness in general. One should remember the qualifying criteria of a depressive episode in DSM-IV quoted above: it should cause "clinically significant distress or impairment in social, occupational, or other important areas of functioning". This is a life-world matter, dependent not only upon how things "really are", but also upon how the person and people around her (family, friends, the doctor) interpret them to be. The question of normality is linked to normative judgments as soon as we enter the field of illness, in contrast to the more scientific-objective domain of disease.

The distinction between illness and disease, however, is certainly not as clear-cut as it might first appear. Diagnosis, especially in psychiatry, but also in many cases of somatic medicine, typically rests on illness criteria, rather than on disease criteria.[16] What should be counted as a too high blood pressure, calling for diagnosis and treatment, ultimately rests on a clinical judgment related to the individual person whose body is being investigated (Svenaeus 2001). What is too high for me could be all right for you, within certain limits. One should be aware that the reason why the domain of the normal is getting narrower every day, is not only that doctors and scientists come to learn more about diseases and become more able to treat them, but also that the companies who manufacture and sell pharmaceutics have a clear interest in pushing the borderlines of what should be treated (Healy 2004). Doctors not only treat a state of the body because it *is* a disease, it *becomes* a disease because it can be treated (Elliott 2003).

We should probably talk more about illness in its own right, instead of constantly slipping into disease-talk. In a way that is exactly what I have been trying to do in the case of Prozac by introducing phenomenology. It is very seductive to talk about serotonin instead of talking about human misery (for doctors as well as patients, not to mention politicians and the representatives of the pharmaceutical companies), but it is not going to get us the whole way, nor even very far, in understanding and helping persons who suffer (Crossley 2003). Do not get me wrong here; I am convinced that SSRIs have helped thousands and thousands of people, who could not have been helped in any other existing way. The phenomenological notion of "bodily resonance" fits well into explaining why the serotonin level could be very important to feelings and being-in-the-world. But our biology needs to be put into this very phenomenological pattern of meaning-constitution, lest we should mystify it and make it into something totally foreign to problems of everyday life. Serotonin talk encourages us to blame our brains rather than our selves and the society we live in (Valenstein 1998). "It is not me who is ill, it is my body". In one way this view on depression (and anxiety disorders) gets it exactly right. The depressed person experiences an *alien* quality, which is present at the heart of her existence and being-in-the-world – the lived body. But this lived body is certainly also *herself*, and not a mere thing.

The ways of the body (biological as well as lived) are not only changed by drugs and other physical influences, such as suffering a stroke, or burning one's hand on the stove, for instance. They are also altered by the feelings and thoughts we have in life. Being depressed might certainly be caused by low serotonin, but this also works the other way around: being bored, sad and anxious might cause the serotonin levels to go down. To raise the serotonin levels in the synapses of the brain by way of an SSRI is a possible cure for depression and anxiety disorders. But it should also be acknowledged that the *belief* that one is raising the serotonin levels by way of an SSRI could lead to relief from illness by itself. According to the Swedish Council on Technology Assessment in Health Care, meta-studies of clinical trials have shown that almost 50 per cent of the effect of SSRIs is placebo or natural recovery (SBU 2004: 197). This is quite a powerful response; the confidence that the medicine will work seems to be almost as important as the medicine itself.

Discussion and concluding comments

In this chapter I have tried to listen to Prozac by way of phenomenology, responding to the invitation of Peter Kramer, made in his much-read book from 1994: *Listening to Prozac*. My strategy has been to understand the relationship between normal feelings and pathology on the phenomenological level, rather than, as Kramer does, asking head on if SSRIs provide a cure that make, not only the ill, but also the healthy, "better than well", by changing their personality traits. My discussion of bodily resonance as a being tuned in different ways, offered above, touches upon this, but it does not give any comprehensive answer to the question whether Prozac is a cure for mental illness, or rather a mood- and personality-enhancer. To be honest, I do not think it is possible to give a straight answer to this question, since the disposition of being attuned in different ways through bodily resonance is not necessarily either an illness or a personality trait. It could be both at the same time, since the lived body is both mine and at the same time alien. I do not fully control the ways of the body; it has a kind of life of its own (autonomous functions), in which it can take on alien qualities (Leder 1990, Svenaeus 2000). And yet the lived body is also me, my point of view on the world, which makes transcendence to the world by way of attunement possible. Bodily resonance is a kind of *activating passivity*. When the passive aspects of embodiment become too foreign and painful, we talk about illness. When the passive aspects are simply the corner-stone of what is me, we talk about personality (melancholic, sanguine, choleric, phlegmatic, or more modern differentiations made by twentieth century psychologists).

We live in a culture in which self-formation is becoming more and more of a mission, instead of something pre-given. This might seem like a paradox: has not recent biomedical progress in areas such as molecular biology and neurophysiology changed our views on personality in a deterministic direction, by which the influence of social environment on the individual has become less important in determining how he is and what he will be? Well, yes and no.

First, the social predetermination of an individual's life plan has loosened up, at least in the minds of people. You are no longer born to be what your father or mother were, and this has changed self-formation radically, especially for women, who are no longer born to be only mothers and wives. This ideal of finding your own way in life, rather than relying on social traditions, has been bred all over the Western world, in the last 50 years or so, by a very influential ideal, summed up by the phrase "the American dream": it is up to yourself and nobody else who you are going to end up being (Elliot 2003).

Second, biomedical developments have not only made it possible to understand and plot the causal networks of our biology in a much more sophisticated way, they have also made it possible to *change* them. This change from chance to choice in the make-up of our bodies will likely have vast effects on future genetic treatments (Buchanan *et al.* 2000), as it has already had in plastic surgery and psychopharmacology (Elliott 2003). Will genetics go down the alley of enhancement (rather than cure for diseases and defects) in the same way plastic surgery already has? And, most important to us here, has psychopharmacology already done so by the aid of SSRIs? Are SSRIs taken to enhance the self, rather than to cure it from diseases and defects?

I have already tried to explain why I think this question is a complex, if not unanswerable, one, since it is far from clear in all cases what is to be taken as a disease or defect, and what is to be taken as an aspect of the self – also from a phenomenological point of view. But let me, as a kind of conclusion, point towards three issues, which I think are necessary to address and understand in order to answer this question. The first issue is that matters of self-enhancement, in the case of SSRIs, are best understood as matters *self-revelation* and *self-adaptation*. Prozac is not a "happy pill", it does not make you cheerful, but it might make you more or less of yourself, so to say. Prozac takes something away that I feel not to be mine (in some cases we prefer to call this "something" a depression, in other cases we should perhaps rather call it a character trait), and in doing this it might be said either to reveal myself the way I really am beneath the disguise of disease, or to help adapt myself to a world in which I could not feel at home the way I was before. Self-creation is always played out and realized in the meaning patterns of society and culture, in which we find ourselves and judge ourselves in different ways. We engage in the norms of what is a normal and good life through our daily activities, striving towards self-fulfillment – authenticity and happiness – together with others. These norms, needless to say, are not only established by psychiatry. They are certainly related to the high-speed, commercial culture of late modern capitalism.

The second point to highlight is that transforming one's life pharmacologically, rather than by way of therapy and will, has become a more powerful and tempting alternative with the advent of SSRIs. It has certainly in many ways become a more *correct* alternative, since self-doubt, self-scrutiny and self-talk cost a lot of money, not only to the individual, but also to society, in terms of treatment and sick leave. And yet, of course, people do not stop talking about their lives, just because they get Prozac. They continue to do so, and now the issue of SSRIs enters these everyday talks. This would be my third and final point: we should start to listen more systematically, not only to Prozac, but also to people talking *about* Prozac, in order to better understand the issues of normativity and authenticity. Is all the talk going on about Prozac an example of what Jürgen Habermas calls the "colonization of the life-world", whereby we medicalize questions properly belonging to the spheres of philosophy, psychology and sociology (Crossley 2003)? Or does it rather offer us a more nuanced account of mental illness and suffering, emphasizing the importance, not only of the brain, but also of the lived body? This is a fascinating task for future research on the SSRI revolution, which I hope to be able to engage in myself.

Notes

1 In 1990 the prescription (sale) rate was 8 DDD (daily defined doses per 1,000 persons each day). In 2000 it was 48 DDD, and in 2004 (statistics available to 30/06/2004) it was 62 DDD (source: www.apoteket.se). It is, of course, hard to know how many of these daily defined doses are actually consumed by the patients. The statistics end when the drugs leave the pharmacy.

2 According to the Swedish Council on Technology Assessment in Health Care, the lifetime incidence of depression is 17–18 per cent (SBU 2004: 73). Given the fact that antidepressants are not only prescribed for depression, but also for a variety of anxiety disorders, 20 per cent of the population could very well be an underestimation. Although I have not carried out systematic comparisons with other countries, it should be pointed out that the Swedish development is by no means unique, possibly not even extreme. In the USA, the cost of antidepressive drugs per citizen is twice as high as in Sweden (statistics from 2001 found at www.nihcm.org and at www.apotektet.se). The total cost of antidepressive medication in the USA in 2001 was 12.5 billion dollars, to be compared with about 0.2 billion dollars in Sweden. The USA has about 293 million citizens; Sweden has about nine million citizens.

3 See Andersson (2003) and Healy (2004) in which the marketing and research strategies of pharmaceutical companies selling antidepressants are critically evaluated and discussed.

4 For the development of antidepressive pharmaceuticals from the time of the Second World War until today, see David Healy's excellent book *The Antidepressant Era* (1997).

5 Indeed, the current expert opinion, based on evaluation of existing clinical trials, is that SSRIs are not more efficient than tricyclics in the treatment of depression. In the case of severe depression, tricyclics even seem to be better than SSRIs (SBU 2004: 191ff.).

6 See www.apoteket.se and www.nihcm.org. In the future, we will probably see new kinds of mood-affecting drugs influencing the levels, not only of serotonin, but also of noradrenaline and other neurotransmitters in the brain. The knowledge of different kinds of receptors for the same substance (there appears to be at least 14 different kinds of receptors for serotonin, for instance) might also lead to new breakthroughs in drug development. Although the big rise in prescriptions of antidepressants in Sweden and other countries has come about through SSRIs, experts are in no way convinced that lack of serotonin is the "magic target" of depression, in any way similar to, for instance, the lack of insulin in diabetes. Matters are far more complex; see, for instance, Healy (1997) and Whybrow (1997).

7 As the title of Peter Kramer's influential book from 1994 urges us to do.

8 In this chapter, the terms "illness" and "disease" are used in accordance with the standard distinction made in the fields of medical philosophy, psychology and sociology between personal experience, on the one hand, and biological processes, on the other.

9 This chapter is inspired by an ongoing empirical research project based on interviews with doctors and patients prescribing and consuming SSRIs. Since I am in the middle of collecting and analyzing the empirical material, it will not be presented in the text. Rather I will aim at analyzing conceptual issues, but the models of understanding I propose have certainly been influenced by the conversations I have enjoyed so far in the project. The literature on depression is certainly vast; for a good introduction with many references see Solomon (2001). See also Elliott and Chambers (2004) for an interesting collection of papers on the SSRI development containing further references.

10 Even if such laboratory tests were developed, the question would of course remain whether they really measured depression, or rather something else.

11 DSM-IV and ICD-10 are to a very large extent compatible, even though the ICD manual lacks the multi-axial assessment, and generally deploys somewhat less fine-tuned diagnostic criteria. Both manuals are diagnostic tools; they do not make any recommendations about treatment. The reason for concentrating on depressive disorders and anxiety disorders below is that the SSRIs have been approved for treatment of these kinds of disorders – as they are specified in DSM and ICD – by regulatory authorities. In Sweden this regulatory authority is "Läkemedelsverket", in the USA it is the "FDA", in Great Britain it is the "MHRA".

12 It should be mentioned at this point that I am certainly not the first one to try to utilize Heidegger's insights in the philosophy of psychiatry. Well-known psychiatrists and psychoanalysts, such as Ludwig Binswanger, Medard Boss, Wolfgang Blankenburg and Jacques Lacan, have developed theories inspired by Heidegger's phenomenology, since the 1930s (Spiegelberg 1972).

13 Heidegger himself, in *The Fundamental Concepts of Metaphysics*, refers to the famous comment by Aristotle, made in the *Problemata*, that all great and creative men have been melancholics (1983: 271). Heidegger writes on the same page that philosophical thinking comes out of basic moods that are characterized by *"Schwermut"* (sadness, melancholy). Anxiety and boredom would thus bear this relationship to sadness and melancholy for Heidegger, a kinship we will return to later in this chapter.

14 Melancholia is the pre-modern expression for depression and depressive personality traits, which disappears around 1900 in the vocabulary of psychiatry. Melancholia, however, has ironically found its way back into contemporary psychiatry. It is found in DSM-IV as a specified type of depression with deep, persistent boredom (2000: 419). In twentieth-century psychiatry, this type of depression has carried many different names – endogenous, vital, biological – all contaminated, however, by etiological hypotheses, which made them unsuitable for the DSM classification. Even more important in this context is the reoccurrence of the old notion of "dysthymia" in DSM, which is similar to the pre-modern notion of melancholia in indicating a certain temperament, or personality type (2000: 376). See Healy (1997) and Kramer (1994).

15 This question is certainly related to the whole field of developmental child psychology and the issue of when the child becomes a subject (ego) in its own right. The reason why very early experiences (being abandoned by the mother, or even being born) are claimed by some researchers to be qualitatively different from later losses in life would be that the child, indeed, at these early stages, was not yet an ego. See Freud (1957b). For more recent theories of child development see Stern (1985).

16 In psychiatry one has tried to get around this (and other) dilemmas, by talking about mental "disorder", instead of disease or illness. But, as should be clear from my paragraph on diagnosis above, what is specified is rather illness- than disease-issues.

References

Andersson, S.J. (2003) *General Practitioners' Conceptions of Depressive Disorders: Associations with Regional Sales of Antidepressive Drugs*, Lund: Faculty of Medicine, Lund University.

Buchanan, A., Brock, D.W., Daniels, N. and Wikler, D. (2000) *From Chance to Choice: Genetics and Justice*, Cambridge: Cambridge University Press.

Crossley, N. (2003) "Prozac nation and the biochemical self: A critique", in S. Williams, L. Birke and G. Bendelow (eds) *Debating Biology: Sociological Reflections on Health, Medicine and Society*, London: Routledge.

DSM-IV (2000) *Diagnostic and Statistical Manual of Mental Disorders*, 4th edn, Washington, DC: American Psychiatric Association.

Elliott, C. (2003) *Better than Well: American Medicine Meets the American Dream*, New York: Norton.

Elliott, C. and Chambers, T. (eds) (2004) *Prozac as a Way of Life*, Chapel Hill, NC: University of North Carolina Press.

Freud, S. (1957a) "Mourning and melancholia", in *The Standard Edition of the Complete Psychological Works of Sigmund Freud*, vol. 14, London: Hogarth.

Freud, S. (1957b) "Inhibitions, symptoms and anxiety", in *The Standard Edition of the Complete Psychological Works of Sigmund Freud*, vol. 20, London: Hogarth.

Fuchs, T. (2000) *Psychopathologie von Leib und Raum: Phänomenologisch-empirische Untersuchungen zu depressiven und paranoiden Erkrankungen* (Psychopathology of Body and Space: Phenomenological and Empirical Investigations of Depressive and Paranoid Disorders), Darmstadt: Steinkopff.

Haar, M. (1992) "Attunement and thinking", in H. Dreyfus and H. Hall (eds) *Heidegger: A Critical Reader*, Cambridge: Blackwell.

Healy, D. (1997) *The Antidepressant Era*, Cambridge, MA: Harvard University Press.

Healy, D. (2004) *Let them Eat Prozac: The Unhealthy Relationship between the Pharmaceutical Industry and Depression*, New York: New York University Press.

Heidegger, M. (1983) *Die Grundbegriffe der Metaphysik: Welt, Endlichkeit, Einsamkeit*, GA 29–30, Frankfurt am Main: Vittorio Klostermann; trans. W. McNeill and N. Walker (1995) *The Fundamental Concepts of Metaphysics: World, Finitude, Solitude*, Bloomington, IN: Indiana University Press.

Heidegger, M. (1986) *Sein und Zeit*, Tübingen: Max Niemeyer; trans. J. Stambaugh (1996) *Being and Time*, Albany, NY: State University of New York Press.

Held, K. (1993) "Fundamental moods and Heidegger's critique of contemporary culture", in J. Sallis (ed.) *Reading Heidegger: Commemorations*, Bloomington, IN: Indiana University Press.

ICD-10 (2004) *International Statistical Classification of Diseases and Related Health Problems*, 2nd edn, Geneva: World Health Organization.

Kramer, P. (1994) *Listening to Prozac*, London: Fourth Estate.

Leder, D. (1990) *The Absent Body*, Chicago, IL: University of Chicago Press.

Merleau-Ponty, M. (1945) *Phénoménologie de la perception*, Paris: Editions Gallimard; trans. C. Smith (1962) *Phenomenology of Perception*, London: Routledge.

Nancy, J.-L. (2003) "Originary ethics", in *A Finite Thinking*, Stanford, CA: Stanford University Press.

SBU (Swedish Council on Technology Assessment in Health Care) (2004) *Behandling av depressionssjukdomar: En systematisk litteraturöversikt*, vol. 1 (Treatment of

Depression: A Systematical Investigation of Research and Literature), Stockholm: SBU.

Solomon, A. (2001) *The Noonday Demon: An Atlas of Depression*, London: Chatto & Windus.

Solomon, R.C. (1993) *The Passions: Emotions and the Meaning of Life*, Indianapolis, IN: Hackett Publishing.

Spiegelberg, H. (1972) *Phenomenology in Psychology and Psychiatry*, Evanston, IL: Northwestern University Press.

Spiegelberg, H. (1982) *The Phenomenological Movement: A Historical Introduction*, 3rd edn, The Hague: M. Nijhoff.

Spitzer, M., Uehlein, F. and Schwartz, M.A. (eds) (1993) *Phenomenology, Language and Schizophrenia*, New York: Springer.

Stern, D.N. (1985) *The Interpersonal World of the Infant*, New York: Basic Books.

Svenaeus, F. (2000) "The body uncanny: Further steps towards a phenomenology of illness", *Medicine, Health Care and Philosophy*, 3: 125–37.

Svenaeus, F. (2001) *The Hermeneutics of Medicine and the Phenomenology of Health: Steps Towards a Philosophy of Medical Practice*, Dordrecht: Kluwer Academic.

Toombs, S.K. (ed.) (2001) *Handbook of Phenomenology and Medicine*, Dordrecht: Kluwer Academic.

Valenstein, E.S. (1998) *Blaming the Brain: The Truth about Drugs and Mental Health*, New York: Free Press.

Whybrow, P.C. (1997) *A Mood Apart: Depression, Mania, and Other Afflictions of the Self*, New York: Basic Books.

Zahavi, D. (1999) *Self-Awareness and Alterity: A Phenomenological Investigation*, Evanston, IL: Northwestern University Press.

Zahavi, D. (2003) *Husserl's Phenomenology*, Stanford, CA: Stanford University Press.

Index

abnormality *see* normality
Adelswärd, V. and Sachs, L. 11, 111, 116, 128
Al-Jader, L.N. *et al.* 116
Aneurysm Support Homepage 145–7, 154
aneurysms: as embodied risk 153–8; intercranial aneurysms 147–8; Internet narratives of 15, 145–7; living with cold aneurysms 152–3; narratives of patients' experiences of 148–52; summary and discussion of 158–60
antidepressive drugs 15, 164, 165
anxiety 168, 169, 171–4, *see also* depressive and anxiety disorders
Armstrong, D. 8, 9–10, 19, 20, 36, 37, 44, 115, 137
Aspegren, K. 21
assisted reproductive technologies 71–2
Atkinson, P. 7, 10
authenticity 171–2

Babes, A. 40
babies: visualisation of during pregnancy 95, 128–31; women's reassessment of risk after birth 131–4
Baggens, C. 96
Baillie, C. *et al.* 116, 118, 120, 135, 136
Bauman, Z. 12
Beauchamp, T.L. and Childress, J.F. 85
Beck, U. 153–4
being-in-the-world (concept of) 170–4
Birke, L. 9, 42, 43, 44
bodily resonance (concept of) 174, 177, 178
the body: and developments in medical technology 19–20, 93; and experiences of brain aneurysms

149–51, 156, 158–9; mood and depressive disorders 173–4, 176–80, *see also* life world
bomb metaphor 15, 157–8
boredom 168, 169, 171–4
Bosch, X. 70
'Brain Aneurysm Narrative-site' 145–7, 154, 159, *see also* aneurysms
Braude, P. *et al.* 72
Bredmar, M. and Linell, P. 11, 111, 117
Britain *see* UK
Broom, A. 20
Brown, N. and Webster, A. 1, 2, 3, 4, 12
Buchanan, A. *et al.* 179

CAM 20
cancer: lay conceptions of 158, *see also* Pap smear tests
Canguilhem, G. 5, 9
Cartwright, L. 42–3, 63
Casper, M.J. and Clarke, A.E. 41
Castells, M. 142–3
Celexa 165
cervical cancer screening *see* Pap smear tests
Charles, C. *et al.* 142
children, genetic disease in 73, 74, 79
choice: and Down syndrome screening 134, 136; 'informed' and Internet access 144; and PGD 81–3, 84–7
Cipramil 165
citalopram 165
City lab 45
Clark, J.A. and Mishler, E.G. 22
Clarke, A.E. and Casper, M.J. 44
classifications *see* cytological classifications
clinical encounter, communication in 7–9
Coburn, D. and Willis, E. 141

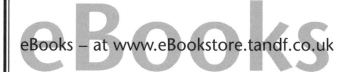